HEAD

C000045702

Other Walker and Company Books
From the People's Medical Society

77 Ways to Beat Colds and Flu

■

67 Ways to Good Sleep

HEADACHES

■

47 Ways to Stop the Pain

Charles B. Inlander
and
Porter Shimer

A *People's Medical Society* Book

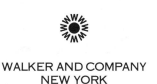

WALKER AND COMPANY
NEW YORK

Copyright © 1995 by People's Medical Society

A note to the reader: The ideas, procedures, and suggestions contained in this book are not intended as a substitute for consulting with your practitioner. All matters regarding your health require medical supervision.

All rights reserved. No part of this book may be reproduced or transmitted in any form or by any means, electronic or mechanical, including photocopying, recording, or by any information storage and retrieval system, without permission in writing from the Publisher.

First published in the United States of America in 1995 by Walker Publishing Company, Inc.

Published simultaneously in Canada by Thomas Allen & Son Canada, Limited, Markham, Ontario

Library of Congress Cataloging-in-Publication Data

Inlander, Charles B.
Headaches : 47 ways to stop the pain / Charles B. Inlander and Porter Shimer.
p. cm.
"A People's medical society book."
Includes index.
ISBN 0-8027-1314-9. — ISBN 0-8027-7473-3 (pbk.)
1. Headache–Popular works. I. Shimer, Porter II. Title.
RB128.I55 1995
616.8′491–dc20

95-20541
CIP

Printed in the United States of America

2 4 6 8 10 9 7 5 3 1

■ CONTENTS

■ INTRODUCTION

"Not tonight, dear, I have a headache."

Those words, believe it or not, are as likely to have been spoken 50,000 years ago as today. Headaches have plagued humanity since the Stone Age, when one remedy was to chisel holes into the skull in hopes of venting pain thought to be caused by demons. Patients often died of the procedure, unfortunately, yet the practice continued for centuries – proof of the desperation to which even the most primitive of headache sufferers could be driven.

Other ancient headache remedies throughout the ages have included draping reptile skins over the head and face, wearing the head of a dead vulture around the neck, rubbing the forehead with a live toad, and drinking tonics concocted of ingredients ranging from cow manure to powdered flies and the sex organs of male beavers.

The search for headache relief, in short, has been an ardent if not always expedient one, and it continues today. Advances in both the understanding and treatment of headaches continue to be made, yet headaches still afflict an estimated 90 percent of Americans to some degree – 20 percent to the point of having to seek medical care. The expense of this epidemic to the American economy, moreover, has in itself been a pain: In terms of sick days and costs for health care and medication, six to eight billion dollars get lost to headache pain every year.

But the good news is that relief *can* be found. Doctors now suspect that chemical imbalances in the brain's delicate pain-sensing mechanisms are at the root of most headaches, and they're finding that these imbalances can be controlled. In *Headaches: 47 Ways to Stop the Pain*, you'll learn not just the latest and most effective methods for relieving headache pain once it strikes, you'll also learn to *prevent* your headaches by determining what triggers them in the first place. It could be something as simple as that hot dog you had for lunch or as complicated as that argument you had over dinner. There may, in fact, be nearly as many causes of headaches as there are people who suffer from them, so the better you can understand your own particular headache problems, the better your chances of solving them are going to be.

Are you up to the challenge?

Good, because it's our mission to help you.

Charles B. Inlander, President
People's Medical Society

HEADACHES

■

1 ∎ Understanding Headaches

"Lord, how my head aches! . . .
It beats as it would fall in twenty pieces."

The nurse, from Shakespeare's *Romeo and Juliet*

If you had only a skull and brain inside your head, it is unlikely you would have headaches, because neither the brain nor the skull is capable in itself of experiencing pain. Only nerves can experience pain, and in the case of headaches, these nerves abide within the face, scalp, and neck and in the brain's protective covering, known as the *meninges*. The type of headache you suffer depends on which of these nerves are being aggravated, and why.

When tense muscles are the source of nerve aggravation—as is the case in over half (some 60 percent) of all headaches—the result is the dull, usually nonpulsating ache of what's known as a muscular-contraction, or tension, headache. If expanded blood vessels are the cause of nerve irritation, a vascular headache occurs, and the pain tends to be sharper and more throbbing, with pain frequently being felt with every beat of the heart. About 30 percent of all headaches are in the vascular category, with migraine and cluster headaches being the most common.

Headaches may even be a combination of the two: tension (muscular-contraction) and vascular. (Only about 10 percent of all headaches are organic—symptoms or side effects of other conditions,

1

such as tumors and head injuries, or diseases like glaucoma. We have more to say about this later in this chapter.)

Some researchers now feel that rather than stressing the distinction between the two general types, we would be more accurate viewing headache pain as a continuum—vascular headaches simply being a more extreme form of the muscular-contraction variety. Recent studies show that certain drugs effective in treating migraines also help relieve tension types, which supports this theory.

It's important to know more about these basic headache types so you can determine which ones might be causing problems for you. Then you'll be able to tailor your own remedial program from the therapeutic tips that follow.

Tension Headaches: When Muscles Make the Ache

Tension headaches, or muscular-contraction headaches, are by far the most common. The accepted theory is that prolonged contraction of muscles in the shoulders, neck, face, or scalp impinges on blood vessels, thereby reducing blood flow. This in turn produces an oxygen shortage within the muscles as well as an unnatural accumulation of pain-producing toxins because blood flow is insufficient to sweep the toxins away. The result: a tension headache, as nerves within the contracted muscles become irritated and communicate this irritation to the brain.

Usually a tension headache begins as a dull, nonpulsating ache that starts at the back of the head and moves forward, eventually creating a feeling of intense pressure at the top of the head or in the forehead or temples (as if you were wearing a hat that's too tight). Frequently muscles of the shoulders and neck also ache, as may the scalp. The pain is usually bilateral, affecting both sides of the head equally.

While most tension headaches subside on their own within a few hours, some can linger for days or even weeks, depending on their causes. Tension headaches usually do not interfere with sleep, however, although some can survive a full night of sleep, being there to greet the sufferer bright and early in the morning. Emotional factors, such as stress, anxiety, and depression, can be contributing causes of tension headaches, as can physical factors, such as eyestrain, poor posture, periods of extended sitting, excessive squinting or jaw clenching, misalignments of the neck or spine, arthritic conditions of the neck or spine, or an injury to the neck or spine, such as whiplash.

Tension headaches are not thought to be an inherited problem, but they do tend to run in families, perhaps because families tend to share many personality traits. If parents deal poorly with stress, for example, their children are apt to do the same. And while some surveys indicate that tension headaches afflict more women than men, many experts believe women are merely more likely to seek medical attention for their headaches than men.

Pain "Referred," But Still Real

If tension headaches originate in the shoulders, neck, or face, why are they usually felt in the head? Referred pain is the culprit. Referred pain is a very complex and not yet fully understood phenomenon. It's thought to result from pain signals getting slightly "crossed" when pain from more than one location must travel to the brain through the same nerve at the same time. This is why damage to the heart during a heart attack can be felt in the arm rather than the chest, and a pinched nerve in the lower back can produce pain in one of the legs. Certain key nerves can get overloaded with pain stimuli, resulting in pain felt somewhere other than its actual site.

In the case of headache pain, according to most experts, such neurological overloads occur mostly within the trigeminal nerve. This is the largest nerve of the head and is responsible for transmitting pain signals to the brain, not just from the muscles of the face and jaws, but also from the sensitive tissues of the forehead, scalp, mouth, throat, eyes, sinuses, and the meninges. Pain signals originating from any of these areas serviced by the trigeminal nerve, therefore, have potential for being felt in any of the other areas, because the pain signals can get mixed during their journey along the same basic nerve "highway."

Pain caused by eyestrain, as an example, can be perceived as pain in the area of the temples. Or pain resulting from eating ice cream too fast, by irritating nerves at the back of the throat, can be perceived as an ache in the area of the forehead.

The trigeminal nerve is not the only one capable of producing referred pain due to sensory overload, however: Several of the major spinal nerves carrying messages to the brain from the muscles of the neck and shoulders also can get their signals crossed. When these muscles tense up, such as during periods of extended immobility or emotional stress, nerves within the muscles become irritated, resulting in pain that can be "referred" to nerves within the temples, forehead, or scalp.

Tension Headaches' Most Common Characteristics

Although symptoms of tension headaches can be similar to those of headaches due to other causes (which we discuss shortly), there are certain key characteristics doctors look for. According to the International Headache Society's Diagnostic Criteria, here are the most common:

■ The pain of a tension headache usually is moderate rather than severe, and steady and dull rather than throbbing and sharp, often described as though the head were being squeezed in a vise.

■ The pain, which can last anywhere from 30 minutes to several days, usually affects both sides of the head equally and may be accompanied by pain or stiffness in the shoulders and/or neck.

■ Periods of prolonged immobility, such as long drives or extended periods of sitting, may bring on pain.

■ The pain is not made worse by continuation of normal physical activity.

■ The pain may be accompanied by a loss of appetite, but not severe nausea or vomiting.

■ The pain often is associated with feelings of depression or emotional stress.

■ The pain generally is not accompanied by other health problems and the sufferer otherwise is usually in good health.

Adapted from the International Headache Society's Diagnostic Criteria and *Freedom From Headaches*, by Joel R. Saper, M.D., and Kenneth R. Magee, M.D., New York: Simon and Schuster, 1981.

Vascular Headaches:
When Blood Vessels Produce the Pain

Abnormal expansion or contraction of blood vessels both inside the skull (on the brain's surface and within its protective covering, the meninges) as well as outside the skull (in the tissues of the face, scalp, mouth, throat, sinuses, and neck) also can cause headache pain. The expansion or contraction of these blood vessels irritates nerves wrapped around the vessels, resulting in the pulsating pain characteristic of vascular headaches.

Migraine headaches are a type of vascular headache, as are the less common but all-too-excruciating type known as cluster headaches, so named for their tendency to occur in groups of four or more in a single day. Also in the vascular category are many headaches caused by certain specific lifestyle triggers, such as eating foods to which the person is sensitive, spending too much time in the sun, overindulging in alcohol, sleeping with bedcovers over the face, skipping meals, or taking certain vasoactive medications for conditions like high blood pressure, angina, and arthritis. These headache triggers are explored in depth in the following chapters.

Migraine Headaches: Classic vs. Common

Migraine headaches, which occur in two forms—"classic" and "common"—are suffered by about 11 percent of the U.S. population. Only about a tenth of all migraine victims have the classic form, where the headache phase of the attack is preceded by 10 to 30 minutes of bizarre sensory disturbances called auras. (This stage does not occur in common migraines.) Vision can become blurred during the aura, or blind spots or even flashing lights may appear. Hearing also can become temporarily impaired, as can speech, muscular control, and balance—the result of a shortage of blood to the brain due to a sudden constriction of the brain's primary arteries. Exactly why this constriction occurs remains in question, but under investigation currently is a brain chemical called serotonin, a potent vasoconstrictor that is found in increasing levels shortly before the aura stage.

The headache phase of a migraine attack is similar for both classic and common migraines. In this stage, the brain's blood vessels undergo a sudden expansion, stretching and irritating nerves wrapped around the vessels, which causes the throbbing pain so characteristic of a migraine attack. Usually the pain–which can last anywhere from 1 to 72 hours–comes on gradually and begins more on one side of the head than the other. It may begin in the area of the forehead, around one of the eyes or temples, or in the vicinity of one of the ears or the jaws. Pain in the muscles of the shoulders and neck also may occur.

The discomfort of a migraine attack can be so encompassing that it involves virtually the entire body. Severe nausea or vomiting may accompany the headache pain, as may diarrhea, dizziness, frequent urination, facial numbness, chills, cold hands and feet, extreme sensitivity to light or noise, mental confusion, and–as in the preheadache phase–difficulties with muscle control and speech. When such attacks finally subside, many victims report–not surprisingly–feeling mentally and physically wiped out for days.

Migraine attacks can vary in severity as well as in frequency and duration. Various factors can trigger migraine attacks; here are some common ones that have been identified:

- dietary sensitivities, especially to alcohol and to foods containing amines or nitrites
- sudden changes in the weather
- physical exertion
- bright or flickering lights
- changes in sleep patterns
- breathing noxious fumes or heavily polluted air
- high altitudes
- low blood sugar
- emotional upsets
- in women, hormonal fluctuations related to menstruation

Who Gets Migraine Attacks?

Research shows that women are more than twice as likely as men to suffer from migraines, with women between the ages of 30 and 49 being especially predisposed. Research also shows that 65 percent of migraine sufferers have a history of the condition in their families.

Whether this is due to genetic inheritance or environmental conditioning remains in question, though probably both factors are at play, most researchers agree.

Writing on the hereditary influence, R. Michael Gallagher, M.D., reports in *Drug Therapy for Headache** that one study found that 46 percent of migraine sufferers had a history of migraine headaches in their families—compared to only 18 percent for sufferers of tension headaches. Yet another study found this association to be even stronger, with 65 percent of migraine patients reporting a close family member to be similarly afflicted. A study involving children with migraines found nearly an 80 percent incidence of the condition in a parent or sibling, says Gallagher.

As to the environmental influence, the executive director of the National Headache Foundation, Seymour Diamond, M.D., explains: "A child watches a parent with migraine and perhaps observes the special treatment the parent gets from the rest of the family. The child then begins to imitate the parent's headache pattern in order to get the same special treatment, and before you know it, the child has a migraine headache that is quite genuine."

Although migraines can begin at any point in a person's life, they usually begin by adolescence, with over half of all migraine sufferers experiencing their first attack by the age of 13. People between the ages of 35 and 45 appear to be most susceptible to attacks. And people whose household incomes are less than $10,000 suffer 60 percent more migraines than those with household incomes of $30,000 or more.

Migraine Headaches' Most Common Characteristics

Although migraine headaches have been known to upset the body to the point of causing tension headaches as a secondary problem, doctors have pinpointed these symptoms in making a migraine diagnosis:

■ The headache affects one side of the head or face more than the other.

■ The headache tends to pound or throb.

---

*New York: Marcel Dekker, 1991.

■ The headache is accompanied by a heightened sensitivity to light and noise.

■ The headache is accompanied by nausea or vomiting.

■ The headache can be severe enough to wake up the sleeping sufferer.

■ The headache is made worse by physical movement, especially bending over.

■ Certain foods seem to trigger the headache (wine, cheese, hot dogs, chocolate, vanilla, citrus fruits, yogurt, or soy sauce, for example), as can going six hours or more without eating.

■ The headache often occurs on weekends, holidays, vacations, or during "letdown" periods following times of unusual excitement or stress.

■ In women, the headache usually occurs during menstruation or a day or two before or after.

■ There is a history of migraine headaches in the sufferer's family.

Adapted from the International Headache Society's Diagnostic Criteria and *Freedom From Headaches*, by Joel R. Saper, M.D., and Kenneth R. Magee, M.D.

Cluster Headaches: "Like a Red-Hot Poker in the Eye"

Cluster headaches also are of the vascular variety but are relatively rare (affecting only about 1 percent of the population, 85 percent of them male). The headaches occur in clusters of several per day for days or even weeks, then suddenly disappear for months or even years. They generally last from 15 minutes to an hour each and are so excruciating they have been known to drive their victims to suicide.

Less is known about the precise biological mechanisms responsible for cluster headaches than about any other headache type. But there is general agreement that they are vascular in nature, and that hormonal imbalances caused by periodic disturbances within the hypothalamus portion of the brain may play a key role.

Particularly important to the pain of cluster headaches seems to be dilation of the carotid artery (the vessel that leads from the heart to the brain via the neck and is the brain's primary source of blood) and irritation to nerves located in the area behind the eye, called the cavernous sinus, which is caused by dilation of a large vein there. Most experts agree that this is why the pain of cluster headaches characteristically strikes the eye area.

Cluster-headache pain may start as a feeling of fullness in one of the ears, but invariably it progresses to an intensely piercing sensation felt behind one of the eyes. Tearing and reddening of the eye, as well as nasal congestion, facial flushing, and sweating are common. The pain has been described graphically by some patients as the feeling of a red-hot poker being pushed through the eye to the point of being embedded in the brain. On other occasions they describe feeling as though their skin were being clawed from their faces and the exposed flesh doused with acid.

Such pain usually affects only one side of the face at a time but may switch to the other side in subsequent attacks, with sufferers frequently pacing about, shouting out loud, or sometimes banging their heads against objects to divert their attention from their pain. Periods of attack tend to be seasonal, with research showing the spring and fall to be the most conducive. Certain lifestyle factors—principally heavy smoking and drinking—appear to increase a person's risk of cluster headaches, but the risk does not show a pattern for being genetically inherited or influenced by upbringing.

Cluster Headaches' Most Common Characteristics

As with migraine headaches, not all cluster headaches exhibit precisely the same symptoms in every sufferer. But some fairly common characteristics have been identified:

■ The headaches occur in groups of between four and eight per day.

■ Once the headaches strike, they continue to do so every day or every other day, for a period of one to three months.

■ The headache sufferer generally is free of headaches except for the cluster episodes.

■ During attacks, nasal congestion or discharge occurs in the nostril on the same side of the face as the pain.

■ During attacks, there is watering of the eye on the same side of the face as the pain.

■ The pain is made worse by bending over.

■ Drinking even small amounts of alcohol can bring attacks on.

Adapted from the International Headache Society's Diagnostic Criteria and *Freedom From Headaches,* by Joel R. Saper, M.D., and Kenneth R. Magee, M.D.

Sinus Headaches: Are They or Aren't They?

Although many people suffer from what they refer to as sinus headaches, Alan M. Rapoport, M.D., and Fred D. Sheftell, M.D., the founders and directors of the New England Center for Headache, in Stamford, Connecticut, report that sinus headaches are actually quite rare. Only about 2 percent of the population has ever suffered from a headache due to true sinus infection. These doctors say that the vast majority of people who categorize their headaches as being caused by sinus infections are in fact experiencing symptoms of a migraine attack, or sometimes a cluster headache, instead.

Migraine and cluster headaches can cause dilation of blood vessels within the sinus cavities, resulting in pain similar to that caused by a sinus infection. There is one key difference, however: Headaches due to true sinus infection are accompanied by a mild to moderate fever, noticeable nasal congestion or discharge, and a feeling of overall debilitation. If headaches are not accompanied by these symptoms, they are probably not due to sinus troubles. If they are, however, a doctor should be seen and he'll probably prescribe antibiotic treatment.

A Word on Women and Headaches

Migraine headaches occur more frequently in women than in men: An estimated 70 percent of migraine sufferers are female (though men may suffer as often as women do from tension-type headaches).

Why this disproportionate susceptibility to migraine headaches among women? Fluctuations in the female hormone estrogen seem to be a potent trigger for migraines. Migraines can be brought on not only by decreases in estrogen (as in the few days before menstruation, or following menopause or hysterectomy) but also by increases in the hormone (as when women take birth-control pills, experience the first trimester of pregnancy, or undergo hormone-replacement therapy following menopause or hysterectomy).

Estrogen's effects vary from woman to woman, however. What worsens one woman's headaches may improve another's. Exactly why these variances exist is unknown, but they are believed to relate to estrogen's effects on how a woman metabolizes serotonin, the brain chemical suspected of being influential in the onset of migraine headaches.

Research also shows that women seek medical care for tension headaches more than men by roughly threefold. But some doctors have been slow to give full credence to women's headache complaints, according to Rapoport and Sheftell.

Organic Headaches: Those That Definitely Need a Doctor

As painful as headaches are, they usually do not signal serious health problems. But there are times when headaches are associated with conditions or diseases that require medical attention. Before embarking on a headache-treatment program of your own, you should see your doctor for the purpose of ruling out serious conditions, including brain tumor, cerebral hemorrhaging (bleeding within the skull), aneurysm (a permanently and abnormally swollen blood vessel within the skull), temporal arteritis (inflammation of arteries in the temples), meningitis (a potentially fatal infection of the brain's protective covering), and glaucoma.

Below are symptoms that could indicate your headaches are of a serious nature. Seek immediate attention, by either calling a doctor or going to a hospital emergency room.

■ Headaches accompanied by neurological problems, such as numbness, weakness, loss of muscular control, or disturbances of vision or speech. (It may be only a migraine, but you could be risking your life by not finding out.)

■ Headaches that increase suddenly in intensity, frequency, or duration. (Again, migraines or cluster headaches can show such symptoms, but it's important to have other, potentially more serious causes ruled out.)

■ Any headache that comes on suddenly and excruciatingly in a fashion you've never experienced before. (Headaches due to a ruptured blood vessel on the surface of the brain may be experienced this way.)

■ Headaches following an injury to the head. (Serious blows to the head may result in blood clots in the brain or injury to the muscles, tendons, nerves or vertebrae of the neck, all of which should be treated by a trained medical professional.)

■ Headaches accompanied by fever, stiff neck, nausea, and vomiting. (Again, be aware that these are symptoms of migraine headaches, but they also could indicate meningitis.)

■ Headaches accompanied by any other unusual symptoms not experienced before, such as fever, shortness of breath, or problems with the eyes, ears, nose, or throat.

■ Headaches accompanied by memory loss and/or confusion—common signs of brain tumor.

While the following symptom may also indicate a serious problem, it does not necessarily require immediate medical intervention. Consult a doctor soon if this symptom persists:

■ Headaches that begin to occur regularly after the age of 50. (Because headaches tend to become less of a problem as we age, all headaches that begin to occur chronically beyond middle age should be checked out. They could be a sign that the brain is not getting enough oxygen due to lung disease, a heart condition, or a vascular disorder, such as hardening or blockage of the arteries.)

Adapted from the International Headache Society's Diagnostic Criteria and *Freedom From Headaches*, by Joel R. Saper, M.D., and Kenneth R. Magee, M.D.

Psychogenic Headaches: Those That Stem From the Mind

"Emotional factors do play an important role in triggering headaches in many people," write Joel R. Saper, M.D., and Kenneth R. Magee, M.D., in their book *Freedom From Headaches*. Some headaches may indeed be psychogenic (emotionally triggered), but even though the cause may be psychological, the effect is clearly real.

Some common pain-producing emotions are extreme or continual stress, worry, or internalized anger, studies show. These emotional states can lead to prolonged contraction of muscles of the face, scalp, shoulders, or neck—and hence a tension-type headache—or dilation of blood vessels in these areas with a vascular headache as the result.

Just as adverse emotional states can produce physical ailments, the reverse can be true: Physical ailments (chronic headaches included) can produce adverse emotional states. The greater the headache pain, the greater the dread and depression associated with it, and the greater the likelihood that even more headaches will ensue.

There are some headaches that exist purely in the mind. Nonorganic headaches (without any discernible physical causes) feel very real but cannot be traced to any adverse biological state. They may be the result of internalized feelings of guilt, anger, depression, anxiety, or fear—the headache can become an embodiment of emotions or past experiences too upsetting to acknowledge, much less openly express. Such headaches characteristically do not respond to medicinal or physical therapies; psychotherapy or some other type of intense psychological counseling usually is required to put them to rest.

2. Causes and Prevention of Headaches

If you suffer from headaches on a regular basis, you have lots of company. Chronic headaches are a problem for an estimated 40 million Americans, and throughout history some very talented and productive people have suffered from recurrent headaches—Charles Darwin, Karl Marx, Thomas Jefferson, Leo Tolstoy, Virginia Woolf, Edgar Allan Poe, and Sigmund Freud, to name just a few.

But significant advances in the understanding and treatment of headaches have been made over the years. Not only can most headaches now be relieved once they strike, many can be prevented from occurring in the first place. The key to conquering headaches is "getting to know them," the experts say—learning which types of headaches you experience and what causes them.

Whether your headaches are only mild and occasional pains or severe and chronic skull slammers, take heart in knowing they can be overcome.

That said, let's look at what the latest research indicates are the best precautionary measures you can take to prevent headaches from striking in the first place. After that, in Chapter 3, we'll look at the most effective ways to relieve headaches when they do occur.

Rule out organic headaches due to potentially serious medical causes.

Anyone who suffers from severe or recurring headaches should first have a medical checkup to rule out the possibility the headaches could be due to a potentially serious health problem. Although very few headaches fall into this organic category, even the slim odds that you may have an organic headache warrant the peace of mind that a medical exam can afford. Here's what you should expect from your headache exam:

■ **A detailed history of your headaches.** You will be asked questions so your physician can determine the type of headaches you're experiencing. Expect the questions to touch on such matters as how the headaches feel, when they occur, their location, their frequency, their duration, and their relation to lifestyle factors, such as diet, alcohol intake, sleep patterns, emotional states, medications you may be taking, and your menstrual cycle if you're a woman. You are also likely to be asked questions regarding your medical history, occupation, hobbies, and personal life to determine which may have some bearing on your headaches.

■ **A thorough physical examination.** The exam should include tests of your neurological and sensory functions in addition to such basics as blood pressure and normal functioning of your heart and lungs.

■ **Urine and/or blood tests.** These tests may be ordered to check for proper functioning of your liver and endocrine (hormonal) system.

■ **X rays, MRI (magnetic resonance imaging, which uses a magnetic field, instead of radiation, to produce detailed, computer-generated pictures of the body), or a CAT scan (a computerized process in which hundreds of x rays are combined into a single picture).** The purpose of these tests: to help rule out the possibility of a brain tumor, cerebral hemorrhage, blood-vessel abnormality, or previous injury to your skull or spine being the cause of your headaches. In certain cases, an electroencephalogram (EEG) also may be requested to test for any abnormalities in the functioning of your brain.

After you have been assured that your headaches are not a symptom of a serious medical condition, you can turn your attention to preventing another headache attack.

 Keep a headache diary.

Because headaches can be caused by so many different factors or combinations of factors, headache experts recommend maintaining a detailed record of the circumstances under which your headaches occur. Seymour Diamond, M.D., executive director of the National Headache Foundation, director of the Diamond Headache Clinic (Chicago), and professor of pharmacology and molecular biology at the Chicago Medical School, suggests keeping a log of your headaches. And in several weeks, you're likely to see patterns emerge regarding the causes of your headaches as well as the relative degrees of success achieved by different methods of prevention and treatment. Your diary should include the following data, Diamond suggests:

- ✔ Date

- ✔ Time of headache onset

- ✔ Time of headache remission

- ✔ Severity of headache (severe, moderate, mild)

- ✔ Foods and beverages consumed prior to headache onset

- ✔ Emotional and/or physical circumstances associated with headache onset

- ✔ Medication taken and amount
      Degree of success achieved

- ✔ Other remedial efforts made
      Degree of success achieved

Medications: When the Solution Becomes Part of the Problem

If you suffer from headaches on a daily or near-daily basis and your usual response is to take a medication to relieve them, here's something that may surprise you: Those pills could be the cause of your problems! Studies show that slightly over half of all chronic headaches—regardless of their type or original cause—eventually become rebound headaches. (See page 19.) They can be caused by prescription and nonprescription medications alike, and they demonstrate a danger that exists with pain-relieving drugs in general. In providing relief unnaturally and temporarily at best, they allow for a deterioration of the mechanisms that, without the drugs, would have a better chance of correcting the situation naturally. The drugs become a crutch, in a sense, allowing the body's natural healing systems to decline. Writing in *The Doctor's Book of Home Remedies*,* the director of the Michigan Headache and Neurological Institute in Ann Arbor, Joel Saper, M.D., explains: "It's like scratching a rash; the more you scratch, the more it itches."

With respect to headaches specifically, pain relievers are believed to "suppress the activity of central serotoninergic pathways concerned with pain regulation, paradoxically making the patient more vulnerable to the return of headache when the analgesic begins to wear off," writes Jerome Walker, M.D., in the November 1993 *Southern Medical Journal.*

 Don't rely continually on headache pills.

How can you know if your own attempts at pain relief are doing more harm than good? "If you have daily headaches and are taking analgesics . . . more than four days a week, you are probably suffering from the analgesic rebound effect," write the founders and directors of the New England Center for Headache, in Stamford, Connecticut, Alan M. Rapoport, M.D., and Fred D. Sheftell, M.D., in their book *Headache Relief.*†

---

*Emmaus, Pa.: Rodale Press, 1990.
† New York: Simon and Schuster, 1990.

MEDICATIONS CAPABLE OF CAUSING THE REBOUND EFFECT

Here's a list, in order of least to most potentially addicting, of pain medications capable of causing the rebound effect (examples of brand names in parentheses):

- acetaminophen (Tylenol)
- acetylsalicylic acid, or aspirin (Bufferin, Bayer)
- nonsteroidal anti-inflammatory drugs, including ibuprofen (Advil)
- butalbital-acetaminophen-caffeine compounds (Esgic, Fioricet, Repan)
- butalbital-acetylsalicylic acid-caffeine compounds (Fiorinal, Lanorinal, Marnal)
- acetaminophen with codeine phosphate (Tylenol with Codeine No. 1 [7.5 mg. of codeine phosphate]; Tylenol with Codeine No. 2 [15 mg. of codeine phosphate]; Tylenol with Codeine No. 3 [30 mg. of codeine phosphate]; Tylenol with Codeine No. 4 [60 mg. of codeine phosphate])
- butalbital-acetylsalicylic acid-caffeine compounds with codeine phosphate
- acetaminophen with synthetic codeine preparations
- acetylsalicylic acid with synthetic codeine preparations
- meperidine (Demerol)
- meperidine with promethazine (Anergan, Phenazine, Phenergan)
- other narcotics

Source: American Family Physician (March 1993).

If you have been taking only over-the-counter medications (e.g., acetaminophen, ibuprofen, aspirin, or naproxen sodium), you should be able to discontinue them without side effects debilitating enough to necessitate professional medical care, Rapoport and Sheftell say. But if you've been taking a stronger prescription drug, particularly one containing codeine, you should consider enrolling at a health-care center or hospital, where you may be prescribed special medications to help alleviate the nausea and worsening of headache pain that frequently accompany the withdrawal process.

Research shows that approximately half of all people suffering from rebound headaches, regardless of the type of original headaches or their causes, experience marked improvement within four weeks of stopping their medications. Even more (85 percent) experience improvement within three months.

Of course, it is best not to fall into the trap of rebound headaches in the first place, the experts agree. Rapoport and Sheftell report that one regular (325 mg.) aspirin tablet (or its equivalent in ibuprofen or acetaminophen) provides all the pain relief you're going to get. The active ingredients are usually absorbed in 15 to 30 minutes and provide relief for two to four hours. Taking any more than this amount is not going to give any more relief and only risks doing more harm than good.

If you have questions concerning the long-term effects of any medication you're taking, check with your doctor.

 Determine if other medications are making your head ache.

Not just headache medications have potential for going adversely to the head, however. Many medications prescribed for other conditions can cause chemical imbalances capable of leading to headache pain, especially migraines. (See pages 22-23.)

The Nutritional Link

"Of the many environmental factors that may trigger headaches, foods and beverages are perhaps the most common," writes Seymour Solomon, M.D., a professor of neurology at Einstein Medical College and the director of the headache unit at Montefiore Medical Center, in New York, and author of *The Headache Book*.*

---

*Mount Vernon, N.Y.: Consumer Reports Books, 1991.

Complicating this fact, however, is that sensitivity can vary according to the amount of the offending food or beverage consumed, and the time of pain onset (some foods may have an immediate effect while the impact of others may be delayed). There's another inconsistency: A food that causes a headache on one occasion may have little or no effect on another, Solomon says. Those variables aside, though, it's important to do your best to:

 ## Avoid foods and beverages that can trigger your headaches.

Studies have shown that foods and beverages containing amines, monosodium glutamate (MSG), nitrites, caffeine, and aspartame have the greatest potential for acting as headache triggers (see page 25). When you track the pattern of your headaches, your headache diary may reveal a dietary connection to one of these.

Amines, including tyramine, are biological substances (produced by the body as well as occurring naturally in certain foods) that are thought to cause headaches in certain people by causing blood vessels on the surface of the brain to constrict and then expand, with headaches occurring in response to the expansion phase. Foods high in amine content should be avoided or consumed in moderation if your headaches seem to be triggered by them.

MSG is a flavor enhancer added to many processed and packaged foods and is thought to cause headaches (plus sweating and tightness in the chest, face, and jaw) in an estimated 10 to 25 percent of the general population. The headaches, which usually occur approximately 15 to 30 minutes after ingesting MSG, are characterized by a pounding in the area of the temples and a tightness in the forehead. The adverse effects of MSG are thought to be caused by a buildup of MSG in the bloodstream as the result of an inability to adequately digest the compound. Beware of foods as potential MSG hosts, and be sure to check ingredient labels to see if it's there. (MSG sometimes hides in a food ingredient called hydrolyzed vegetable protein, which can consist of as much as 30 percent MSG.)

Nitrites have been used for centuries not just to preserve meats but also to give them their distinctly "cured" taste and an appetizing

(continued on page 24)

COMMON HEADACHE-CAUSING MEDICATIONS

If you're taking a medication not listed but suspect it may be contributing to your headache problems, check with your doctor. (Examples of brand names are in parentheses.)

■ **Birth-control pills**

■ **Drugs to treat high blood pressure**
  ✔ captopril (Capoten)
  ✔ clonidine (Catapres)
  ✔ hydralazine (Apresazide, Apresoline)
  ✔ labetalol (Normodyne, Trandate)
  ✔ metoprolol tartrate (Lopressor)
  ✔ minoxidil (Loniten, Rogaine)
  ✔ nifedipine (Adalat, Procardia)
  ✔ prazosin (Minipress)
  ✔ propranolol (Inderal)
  ✔ reserpine (Serpasil)

■ **Drugs to treat angina**
  ✔ isosorbide dinitrate (Isordil, Sorbitrate)
  ✔ nifedipine (Adalat, Procardia)
  ✔ nitroglycerin (Nitrogard, Nitrostat)
  ✔ verapamil (Calan, Isoptin)

■ **Drugs to treat stomach ulcers**
  ✔ cimetidine (Tagamet)
  ✔ ranitidine HCl (Zantac)

■ **Narcotics**
  ✔ propoxyphene (Darvon, Dolene, Doraphen, Doxaphene, Profene, Pro Pox, Propoxycon)
  ✔ oxycodone with acetaminophen (Percocet, Tylox)
  ✔ hydrocodone bitartrate with acetaminophen (Vicodin)
  ✔ meperidine (Demerol)
  ✔ hydromorphone (Dilaudid)
  ✔ morphine (Astramorph, Duramorph, Roxanol)

(continued on next page)

(continued)

- ■ **Nonprescription pain relievers (aspirin, acetaminophen, ibuprofen, naproxyn sodium) if taken more than twice a week**

- ■ **Nonsteroidal anti-inflammatory drugs (NSAIDs)**
  - ✔ diclofenac (Voltaren)
  - ✔ ibuprofen (Advil, Medipren, Midol, Motrin, Nuprin)
  - ✔ indomethacin (Indameth, Indocin)
  - ✔ ketoprofen (Orudis)
  - ✔ naproxen (Naprosyn)

- ■ **Others**
  - ✔ corticosteroids: for treatment of skin problems, asthma, and arthritis*
  - ✔ dipyridamole (Persantine): for prevention of blood clots
  - ✔ ephedrine HCl (Primatene): for treatment of asthma, bronchitis, and emphysema
  - ✔ estrogen supplements: for birth control as well as for treatment of symptoms of menopause. They may also be used in the treatment of breast cancer and prostate cancer and to help prevent osteoporosis in women after menopause.*
  - ✔ griseofulvin (Fulvicin, Grifulvin, Grisactin): for treatment of fungal infections of the skin, hair, and nails
  - ✔ isotretinoin (Accutane): for treatment of acne
  - ✔ phenothiazines: for treatment of anxiety and other emotional disorders*
  - ✔ piroxicam (Feldene): for treatment of arthritis
  - ✔ trimethoprim/sulfamethoxazole (Bactrim, Cotrim, Septra): for treatment of urinary-tract infections

*Too many subcategories of these drugs exist to list them all here. Check with your pharmacist to find out if a drug you're taking is among these types.

pink or reddish color. They are thought to cause headaches in people sensitive to them by causing an inordinate expansion of blood vessels on the surface of the brain as well as in the areas of the face and scalp. Common enough to be called "hot-dog headaches" (in honor of that especially nitrite-rich item), the headaches generally are experienced as a throbbing pain in the temples within 30 minutes of nitrite ingestion.

As with amines, caffeine increases risk of headaches not by its immediate effect—which is to cause blood vessels on the surface of the brain to constrict—but rather by a secondary effect that causes these blood vessels to expand as the caffeine wears off. Studies show that as little as 435 mg. of caffeine a day can cause this rebound effect, with headaches beginning on day one and lasting as long as six days following caffeine abstention. Such headaches caused by caffeine withdrawal generally are throbbing in nature and usually are made worse by physical exertion.

According to a recent survey by the Centers for Disease Control and Prevention, the artificial sweetener aspartame (marketed since 1981 as NutraSweet and Equal) may be the latest of dietary triggers of headaches. In a study done in 1989, 11 percent of a group of migraine sufferers reported aspartame to be a significant headache trigger. Be on the lookout for it in diet soft drinks, chewing gum, and many low-calorie ice creams and desserts.

 ### Don't skip meals.

Going more than six hours without eating can be a powerful headache trigger even in people not normally headache-prone. Skipping meals can bring on headaches by allowing blood-sugar (glucose) levels to drop too low. This causes blood vessels responsible for getting glucose to the brain to constrict in an attempt to increase the speed of blood flow to the brain—a process that sets the stage for a hunger headache. Not only can the constriction itself cause headache pain, as nerves affected by the constriction become irritated, but the compensatory expansion that inevitably follows this constriction also can cause pain.

The key to avoiding this yo-yo effect is not to let blood sugar drop too low in the first place. For that reason, it may be better to eat four

POSSIBLE HEADACHE TRIGGERS

Foods Containing Amines

Cheese (excluding cream and cottage cheeses)
Vinegar or foods containing it (e.g., relishes, cole slaw, pickled items, mustard, ketchup, and salad dressings)
Organ meats (e.g., liver, kidneys, and sweetbreads)
Pork
Smoked meats and fish
Spinach
Citrus fruits
Bananas
Figs
Plums
Pineapples
Raisins
Avocados
Beans (lima, kidney, soy, and others)
Nuts
Onions
Chocolate
Cream, sour cream, and yogurt
Foods containing yeast extracts (found in certain prepared foods, such as soups)
Alcoholic beverages (especially red wines)

Foods Containing Monosodium Glutamate (MSG)

Chinese foods (restaurant as well as packaged)
Instant and canned soups
Dry-roasted nuts
Processed meats
Self-basting turkeys
Instant gravies
Many TV dinners
Some potato and corn-chip snacks
Many packaged tenderizers and seasonings

Foods Containing Nitrites

Canned hams	Salami	Bacon
Corned beef	Bologna	Pepperoni
Hot dogs	Sausage	Smoked fish

Beverages Containing Caffeine

Coffee, per eight-ounce cup:
  Brewed, 80 to 120 mg.
  Instant, 66 to 100 mg.
Tea, per eight-ounce cup:
  Leaf, 30 to 75 mg.
  Bag, 42 to 100 mg.
  Instant, 30 to 60 mg.
Cocoa, per eight-ounce cup:
  Up to 50 mg.
Cola, per eight-ounce glass:
  15 to 30 mg.
Mountain Dew, per 12-ounce glass: 55 mg.

or five small meals throughout the day rather than two or three large ones, doctors agree. Also try to avoid foods exceptionally high in sugar, as they can drive blood sugar so high that the body responds by driving it back down too far via an inordinate release of insulin from the pancreas.

 ### Have a healthy before-bed snack.

If headaches upon awakening in the morning are a problem for you—the possible result of blood-sugar levels dropping too low during the night—a small before-bed snack high in protein often can help: perhaps a glass of milk, some cottage cheese, a small turkey sandwich, or a piece of hard cheese (provided you're not sensitive to any of these foods).

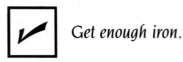 ### Get enough iron.

Iron deficiency can increase headache risk by reducing the blood's ability to carry oxygen, thus partially suffocating virtually every oxygen-dependent cell in the body. Generalized fatigue is a common symptom, but so are headaches, as blood vessels begin to dilate more than normal to make up for the oxygen shortage. Numerous medical conditions can lead to iron deficiencies (blood loss due to hemorrhoids, for example, or peptic ulcer, hiatal hernia, bowel cancer, or diverticulosis). Other conditions, such as heavy menstrual periods, pregnancy, lactation, excessive exercise, and excessive use of aspirin (common in chronic headache sufferers, unfortunately), can also lead to iron deficiency.

After having a checkup to rule out a potentially more serious cause of iron deficiency, you should be sure you're getting enough of the mineral in your diet. Men need at least 10 mg. a day of iron while women require 18 mg. daily, yet many of us fall short of these quotas, especially women during their reproductive years. Lean meats are a good source, as are iron-fortified cereals, green leafy vegetables, fish, beans, raisins, tofu, and eggs.

Vitamin C increases your body's ability to absorb iron, so eat ample amounts of citrus fruits and fresh vegetables. Taking a daily iron supplement also may be a good idea.

 ## Be sure you're getting your B vitamins.

In addition to being important for proper functioning of the nervous system, and thus helping the body deal with emotional stress, the B vitamins aid in the metabolism of carbohydrates. So they can help prevent hypoglycemia (low blood sugar), which is known to bring on headaches in some people. No wonder, therefore, that research shows disproportionately large numbers of migraine sufferers are deficient in these important nutrients.

Making matters worse is that caffeine, alcohol, birth-control pills, and stress are known to deplete the body of B vitamins. In fact, according to George Briggs, Ph.D., and Doris Calloway, Ph.D., of the University of California at Berkeley, more Americans are deficient in vitamin B_6 (pyridoxine) than in any other nutrient. While current RDAs (Recommended Dietary Allowances) for B_6 are 2 mg. for men and 1.6 mg. for women, surveys show that intakes average only 1.87 mg. and 1.16 mg. for males and females respectively.

Although research points especially to the importance of adequate intakes of B_6 and B_3 (niacin) in preventing headaches, it's best to get the entire complex of the B vitamins because the different types complement one another in their similar yet slightly different metabolic actions. This means getting B_1 (thiamine), B_2 (riboflavin), B_{12} (cobalamin), folate, biotin, and pantothenic acid. You can do this either by taking a good B-complex vitamin supplement or by making sure to include a wide variety of B-rich foods in your diet. Broccoli, spinach, green peas, potatoes, whole-grain cereals and breads, wheat germ, liver, eggs, orange juice, peanuts, tuna fish, and brewer's yeast are your best sources.

Healthy Habits Ward Off Headaches

Headaches may be felt only in the head, but factors affecting the entire body can play a contributing role in their development. A healthy lifestyle, therefore, is of great importance in keeping headaches at bay. Heed the following advice with that in mind:

 Stay as regular as possible with your sleep.

Certain headaches (principally migraines and cluster headaches) can be triggered by changes in sleep habits; so sticking to a regular sleep schedule can help prevent their onset, says Pradeep K. Sahota, M.D., of the University of Missouri Medical School. Writing in the *Headache Newsletter,* Sahota recommends that people:

■ Go to bed and arise at the same times every day, weekends especially.

■ Get an adequate amount of sleep each night (between six and eight hours).

■ Get enough physical activity each day to promote restful sleep.

■ Consult your doctor or a sleep clinic if you have chronically had trouble sleeping.

 Adopt good sleeping posture and good bedding.

Best posture is to sleep on your back, not stomach, with a small, loosely filled feather or synthetic-particle pillow that can adapt easily to the shape of your head, says David F. Fardon, M.D., an orthopedic surgeon with the Knoxville Orthopedic Clinic and author of *Free Yourself From Neck Pain and Headache.** "Use of more than one pillow or a large, springy foam pillow may put too much forward push on the head without giving enough support to the natural curve of the neck." Special cervical pillows can be worth their cost, he says, as can quality mattresses.

---

*Englewood Cliffs, N.J.: Prentice-Hall, 1983.

Don't feel you need to go to the expense of a special "orthopedic" mattress, however, he says. As long as your mattress is firm, comfortable, and not sagging, and it's supported by an adequate box spring, it should be treating your back, neck, and head just fine.

 ## Get enough exercise.

Regular physical activity can help prevent headaches (vascular as well as tension types) by virtue of its effects on many of the biological as well as psychological mechanisms known to be headache triggers, says Seymour Solomon, M.D., director of the headache unit at Montefiore Medical Center. Simply by getting between 20 and 30 minutes of aerobic exercise (such as jogging, brisk walking, cycling, or swimming) three to four times a week, most people can boost their resistance to headaches to a significant degree, according to Solomon.

This isn't to say you should exercise during a headache attack, especially if you find it makes your pain worse—usually the case with migraines. Tension and cluster headaches, on the other hand, often can be relieved by physical exertion, so let your experience be your guide. Such acute responses aside, research shows that aerobic exercise done regularly can reduce both the frequency and severity of headaches in most people in the following ways:

- by improving the circulatory system, thus increasing oxygen flow and waste removal within tissues involved in headache pain

- by making blood vessels more elastic, and hence more accustomed to vascular expansions and contractions that might otherwise cause headache pain

- by strengthening muscles responsible for good posture, thus reducing strain on the shoulders, neck, and back

- by increasing levels of pain-relieving chemicals within the body (called endorphins and enkephalins), which have the power to relieve headache pain naturally

- by reducing muscular as well as psychological tension known to trigger headaches

- by elevating mood, thus combating any depression or anxiety that might be playing a role in headache pain

- by helping to promote deeper and more restful sleep, thus eliminating chronic fatigue, which is known to be a headache contributor

- by instilling greater confidence and feelings of control over one's life in general, thus reducing feelings of hopelessness that commonly accompany chronic headache pain

 Don't overdo exercise.

Exercise often gives you a headache, you say, even if you're headache-free at the start? Then you could be overdoing it. Or you could be one of those select few for whom exercise is, in fact, a headache trigger. "Exercise is a two-edged sword in its relationship to headaches," writes Seymour Diamond, M.D., in *Your Patient and Fitness* (May/June 1991). "Whether exercise is appropriate in headache management depends on the type of headache and the patient's individual circumstances," he says.

"About 10 percent of all headache sufferers have exertional aspects to their headaches," Diamond contends. The headaches tend to follow strenuous athletic endeavors like running and weight train-ing, but also can be caused by more routine activities like bending, coughing, sneezing, sexual intercourse, and straining at stool.

Exertional headaches occur most frequently after the age of 40 and in men more than in women. Because such headaches can be dangerous if due to an underlying organic disorder, they definitely should be checked out by way of a thorough medical exam. Then, if no underlying disorder is discovered, simply taking an analgesic several hours prior to exercising usually is effective in preventing or at least ameliorating exertional-headache onset.

Remember, though, to check with your doctor before beginning any exercise routine.   •

Lose weight to diminish headaches.

Yes, excess pounds, especially if they're around the middle, can contribute to headaches, says Fardon, of the Knoxville Orthopedic Clinic. "Excess abdominal fat contributes to the slouched, slumped, head-forward posture that causes much neck, shoulder and head pain," he writes in *Free Yourself From Neck Pain and Headache*. "And the extra fatigue caused by carrying too much weight around can further aggravate the pain."

This isn't to say that obesity is a primary cause of headaches or that weight loss can stop headaches directly, Fardon concedes. Weight loss can help, however, especially if it's achieved slowly and healthfully and in conjunction with other headache-reducing strategies, such as stress control, good nutrition, and regular exercise. Try to "crash" those pounds off and you stand only to make your headaches worse, Fardon warns.

 ## If you smoke, quit.

Many smokers with migraine headaches report improvement when they quit. Tobacco smoking causes blood vessels leading to the brain to dilate (causing headache) to make up for the reduced amount of oxygen the blood of a smoker is able to carry, so quitting smoking restores the blood's oxygen-carrying capacity. Quitting smoking also can help alleviate headaches by helping to reduce the coughing frequently associated with the habit. Less coughing means less strain on the muscles and disks of the neck, as well as less pressure within the blood vessels of the head, which can rise dramatically with each cough. (Quitting smoking can sometimes worsen headaches, but this initial phase usually passes for most people within about a week.)

Heading Off Headaches on the Job

Could it be your job that's making your head ache? If you're working under physically and/or emotionally uncomfortable circumstances, yes. Take these precautions to keep your job as headache-free as possible.

 Stretch frequently and take regular breaks.

Tight muscles, especially in the areas of the shoulders and neck, are a common cause of tension headaches. Stretch frequently during the day to keep these muscles loose—particularly when you're feeling tense or stressed. A simple stretching routine often can help prevent tension-headache onset. Try the following stretch (called the "neck roll") while standing with your feet shoulder-width apart and breathing deeply and slowly. For maximum benefit, the series of maneuvers should take you about five minutes.

Here's how to do it: Let your chin drop slowly to your chest and let it hang there for several seconds. While breathing deeply, roll your head to the right, trying to touch your shoulder with your ear. Hold this position for several seconds, then roll your head forward, then left to your left shoulder, pausing again. When you begin to feel loose, start slowly moving your head in this rolling fashion (keeping your head forward), first to the right for three to five revolutions, then an equal number of times to the left. Finish the stretch (still breathing deeply) by raising your shoulders up in an attempt to make them touch your ears, then dropping them slowly. Repeat five times.

It is very important to take breaks at least every two hours to walk and stretch. (If you find yourself being reprimanded by a supervisor, argue that your productivity will be gaining rather than waning from your efforts.)

Adopt proper sitting habits and use a proper chair.

The human body was not designed to spend hours on end in a fixed position, yet that's what all too many of our jobs in this modern world require. Extended periods of immobility decrease blood flow to the muscles, resulting in a buildup of metabolic waste products that can irritate nerves within the muscles being affected. If these buildups occur in the muscles of the shoulders, back, or neck, headaches can result, as the muscles relay their discomfort to nerves in the sensitive tissues of the face, head, and scalp.

The solution: Sit in a posture as orthopedically correct as possible in a chair as orthopedically correct as possible, says Fardon. Your back should be straight, with your feet firmly planted on the floor, and your head should be held upright rather than thrust forward like that of a turtle looking out of its shell. Further, your chair should be a firm but well-padded one with good support in the lumbar region of your lower back and arm rests for helping to take strain off the muscles of your shoulders and neck.

 ## Don't let your computer give you a headache.

Staring into a computer screen for extended periods can bring on headaches by causing eyestrain. You can minimize this risk, however, by taking five-minute breaks at least every one or two hours, according to experts.

Try to move to a place where the lighting is different from your computer work area, and do the neck-roll exercise we just described to loosen tight muscles of your shoulders and neck. To give your eyes an especially effective reprieve during this break, remove your glasses or contacts, if you wear them, and cover your eyes with your palms, Fred D. Sheftell, M.D., says. Gaze into this darkness for 30 seconds, then close your eyes before removing your hands and slowly reopening your eyes.

Avoid chemical causes of headaches.

Numerous chemical substances encountered in the workplace, home, or workshop–by causing abnormal constriction and/or expansion of blood vessels–also can trigger headaches. Chief among them are:

- organic solvents (e.g., paint thinners and removers)
- paint
- gasoline
- epoxy and other glues
- carbon monoxide from automobiles or faulty home-heating systems
- air pollution from industrial plants
- formaldehyde (present in foam-type insulation and some carpeting)
- garden fertilizers containing nitrates
- tobacco smoke
- strong perfumes

It's best to avoid these potential headache triggers entirely, of course, but if that's not possible, keep exposures as short as possible and be sure the areas in which exposures occur are well ventilated. In the case of high carbon-monoxide levels due to a faulty home-heating system, have your system checked by a heating specialist, because the colorless and essentially odorless gas can be difficult to detect on your own.

Pain-Free-Travel Tips

Travel can be friendly or it can be fiendish for the head. The key is to keep yourself as relaxed and comfortable as possible, whether you're traveling by car, bus, boat, or plane, the experts say. The following tips can help.

Take breaks on long car, train, and bus trips.

Just as sitting at a desk for extended periods can lead to headaches by causing irritation within the muscles of the shoulders, back, and neck, so can sitting behind a steering wheel or in the passenger seat or on a train or chartered bus for hundreds of miles on end. If you're driving, stop every two hours and go for a brief walk and stretch the muscles of your shoulders and neck, using the neck roll described earlier.

If you're on a bus or train that does not stop at comfortable intervals, walk the aisles if you have to, doing the neck roll periodically in between. Also carry a small pillow to place behind your head to help support your neck.

 ## Take these steps to fly less painful skies.

Air travel can be hard on the head for several reasons, says Charles F. Ehret, Ph.D., a senior scientist with the U.S. Department of Energy, in Argonne, Illinois, and author of *Overcoming Jet Lag.** Changes in atmospheric pressure due to rapid rises and falls in altitude, dehydration caused by the stale dry air of most commercial jetliners, prolonged periods of immobility, sleep disruption, and anxiety—all can be headache triggers and make the skies seem very unfriendly indeed.

Ehret and other headache experts offer this advice for making air travel a much more amicable experience:

■ As with car, train, or bus travel, take along a small pillow to place between your seat and the back of the lower part of your head to help take strain off the muscles of your neck.

■ Move around as much as possible. You can do this by walking up and down the aisles, doing deep knee bends in the back of the plane or in the restroom, pressing your hands together in front of your chest, and/or doing the neck-roll exercise.

---

*New York: Berkley Publishing, 1987.

■ Avoid alcoholic beverages. Whatever you think they might do for your "nerves," they're only going to compound the problem of dehydration associated with air travel. Drink fluids, and plenty of them, but make them fruit juices, water, or soft drinks—not several of those four-dollar martinis.

■ Chew gum during takeoffs and landings. It can help your ears "pop" and hence prevent those excruciating buildups of pressure within the sinuses that can occur when planes rapidly rise and descend.

■ Eat as healthfully as possible on your flight. As bad as your air "fare" may be, better to eat it than risk a hunger headache by abstaining. Do opt for the least digestively challenging items being offered, however. Low-fat, not overly spicy dishes are best. And be especially wary of those packets of dry-roasted nuts. They contain hefty amounts of a type of amine (tyramine) known to be a common trigger.

■ Get some exercise upon arriving. Once your feet are back on the ground, get them moving, and preferably in some open air, advises Frank Furtado, athletic trainer for the Seattle Supersonics professional basketball team. Exercise can help rid your body of metabolic waste products that have built up during your flight, as well as help stretch and reoxygenate cramped muscles.

Headaches Caused by the Environment

As with food, the air we breathe can be a potent headache trigger, as can exposure to extreme temperatures, sudden changes in the weather, and too much exposure to the sun. Consider adopting these headache-preventing strategies with that in mind.

 Avoid long periods in the sun.

Skin-cancer risks aside, excessive exposure to direct sunlight (especially during the summer between the hours of 10 A.M. and 3 P.M.) can cause dehydration to the point of drying up fluids responsible for cushioning the spinal cord and brain. The result is a headache, as blood vessels begin to rub ruefully on surrounding tissue. Add a case of tense facial muscles caused by prolonged periods of squinting and you can have a headache extraordinaire – one entirely avoidable, however, simply by staying out of strong sunlight in the first place.

Protect yourself if avoiding the sun is not possible.

If you must spend extended periods in the sun, for whatever reason – maybe your job requires it, for example – protect yourself by wearing a wide-brimmed hat and sunglasses and drink plenty of liquids (nonalcoholic) to keep yourself adequately hydrated. (Sorry, but no piña coladas or frosty beers allowed, because alcohol acts as a diuretic, robbing the body of water required for the metabolism of alcohol.)

Keep enough "negative ions" in your life.

Ions are electrically charged particles in the air – charged either positively or negatively – and are suspected of playing a role in some headaches. In natural environments, the ratio of positive to negative ions is an ideal five to one. But in our more civilized settings – replete with concrete, asphalt, steel, glass, linoleum, vinyl, and central heating and air-conditioning – this ratio can shift. More positive ions are produced, with effects on human health, unfortunately, being decidedly negative. Dizziness and headaches are two of the more common symptoms experienced – problems, according to some estimates, for as much as 25 percent of the population.

Can an overly "positive" environment be avoided, short of moving to Peru? Yes, contends Jonathan V. Wright, M.D., a physician and former columnist for *Prevention* magazine. Devices capable of mechanically producing negative ions have been developed, but short of investing in one of those, you might try the following, Wright says:

■ Avoid wearing synthetic fabrics, which tend to attract positive ions in the form of static electricity. Opt for natural fabrics instead, such as cotton, wool, linen, and silk.

■ Try to go "natural" with your home furnishings as well, using natural rather than synthetic fabrics for draperies, carpeting, slipcovers, and bedspreads.

■ Keep plenty of plants in your home, especially ferns and evergreens, which have an affinity for attracting negative ions.

■ Keep a good circulation of air in your home, with either open windows or fans.

■ Take frequent showers or become a frequent swimmer. (Moving water is known to be a potent producer of negative ions.)

■ Go for regular jogs, walks, or bike rides in the country or drop the top of your convertible if you've got one. (The movement of air, the cleaner the better, also helps create negative ions.)

■ Try to avoid prolonged periods in artificially climate-controlled environments, such as office buildings and department stores, in which negative ions tend to run short.

Be on the lookout for prestorm, weather-related headaches.

Not just our artificial environment can boost positive-ion concentration, however. A dramatic increase in positive-ion concentration frequently accompanies the drops in barometric pressure that precede storms, according to studies by Felix Sulman, M.D., of Hebrew University, in Jerusalem. (Similar increases accompany such world-famous winds as the Santa Ana winds of Southern California, the desert winds of Arizona, the Chinook winds of Canada, and the Autun winds of France, to name just a few, Sulman says.)

Obviously you can't prevent such changes in barometric pressure, but you can prepare for them by taking a nonprescription pain reliever (in moderation, of course) when weather reports forecast a storm front on the way.

Avoid high altitudes.

Especially for sufferers of migraine headaches, high altitudes can trigger attacks due to the decreasing amounts of oxygen available the farther they travel from sea level. Blood vessels responsible for carrying oxygen to the brain expand in an attempt to compensate for the shortage, and bingo—a headache as the expanded vessels irritate neighboring nerves.

Altitudes capable of producing such results vary from person to person, but airline travel and trips to high-altitude mountain resorts are two fairly certain aggravations in those who are susceptible.

Headaches and the Mind-Body Connection

Studies show that the connection between emotional duress and headaches is a strong one. As many as half of all chronic headaches are thought to be due in part to depression, in fact, and certainly the stresses of daily living add heavily to that. Here are some strategies for preventing headaches by defusing some of the emotional factors that can trigger their onset.

 ## Stay "connected" with family and friends.

Good relationships can be good preventive medicine against headaches, according to a study reported in the March 1993 issue of *Headache*. Directed by Paul R. Martin, Ph.D., of the University of Western Australia, in Nedlands, the study compared the social lives of a group of 28 chronic headache sufferers (people averaging at least one headache per week for the previous year) with those of a similar group of 28 people who were relatively headache-free (experiencing less than one headache per month during the previous year). A significant difference was found. Not only did the headache group report having fewer numbers of social relationships (with both family members and friends), they also rated the quality of these relationships to be inferior to those reported by the nonheadache group.

Decreased social life of people in the headache group could have been a result of their headaches. (It's hard to be likeable when you feel miserable.) Then, too, a lack of social support could be a stressor in itself, one capable of increasing headache risk, the researchers said. Feelings of loneliness or abandonment can be subtle but nonetheless powerful headache triggers for people who may already be predisposed biologically.

Either way, headache sufferers would do well to look after the health of their social lives as much as their bodies, says Martin, and doctors treating headache patients should be aware of this potential influence of social factors as well.

 ### Reduce your levels of stress.

How important is stress in the development of headaches? David E. Glass, M.D., associate professor of psychiatry and neurology at the UCLA School of Medicine, answers that question this way: "It has been my personal observation that until a patient's emotional house is in order, headaches will often continue. There is little doubt that emotional stress, either acute or chronic, renders many patients more vulnerable."*

As for the specific types of stressors that seem to be the most potent headache instigators, Bernard H. Shulman, M.D., director of psychiatric services at the Diamond Headache Clinic, in Chicago, cites "the stress of living in an unhappy marriage, of working for a critical and intimidating superior, of long hours of frustration, or of family unhappiness."† Stressors that are chronic and unrelenting, in other words, seem to be the greatest headache poisons.

Also common among chronic headache sufferers are certain personality traits that tend to make their perception of environmental stresses even greater. Shulman cites tendencies toward perfectionism, high ambition, conscientiousness, emotionality, difficulty in dealing

---

*Headache Quarterly (March 1992).
† Headache Quarterly (April 1993).

with ambiguity, strong needs for social approval, and altruism frequently accompanied by feelings of guilt for not being altruistic enough. The result: chronic stress, as these people "are less able to protect themselves against excessive demands from others, feel too guilty to avoid onerous tasks, and will give in rather than engage in unpleasant confrontations,"* Shulman says.

So is the key to avoiding stress-induced headaches simply to become more of an SOB? To a degree, yes, therapists concur. The more you can free yourself from the chronic need for the approval of others, the more you can begin to understand, develop, and approve of yourself. Here is some advice, gleaned from a variety of experts, for doing just that:

■ Don't be afraid to speak your mind. Whatever stress this might cause you initially is usually preferable to the accumulation of stress (in the form of frustration and resentment) if you do not.

■ Accept your limits. The sky may be the limit, but that doesn't mean you should feel guilty for not being able to fly. Work to the best of your ability and try to feel satisfied with that alone.

■ Stop trying to please everybody. Inevitably you'll wind up cheating yourself in some way if you do.

■ Think positively. Whenever you're bothered by what you don't have, remind yourself of what you do.

■ Laugh and smile more often. Research shows that by causing the release of natural mood elevators called endorphins, it can make you feel better even if you don't mean it.

■ Cry more often. Many therapists say it's the most potent stress reliever going, rivaled only by a good, loud scream when the time is right.

■ Get up earlier. Many headache-prone people find they can reduce their headaches simply by getting up 10 to 15 minutes earlier in the morning. The few minutes of sleep lost wind up being well worth it in terms of feeling more on top of things all day long.

---

* *Headache Quarterly* (April 1993).

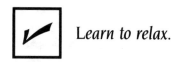 *Learn to relax.*

Because tense muscles, especially in the areas of the shoulders and neck, are a common cause of many headaches, making concerted efforts to relax these muscles can be an effective preventive strategy, studies show. According to a 1994 report in *Behavioral Medicine*, headache patients taught the relaxation techniques discussed below experienced improvements averaging over 50 percent—results slightly superior to those achieved by taking drugs for migraine and tension headaches alike!

FIVE RELAXATION OPTIONS

Find a relaxation technique that best suits your own particular lifestyle and temperament. Although more time consuming than swallowing a few pills, these drug-free techniques are beneficial and far less risky.

■ Progressive Relaxation

Developed by Dr. Edmond Jacobson back in 1929, the technique has withstood the tests of time. It involves tensing and then relaxing the body's muscles "progressively," or one group at a time. The goal is to teach the body how a relaxed muscle actually feels (in contrast to a chronically contracted one) so that the relaxed state might be more easily achieved during times of stress. Before performing the technique, you should first loosen any tight clothing and remove all eyeglasses, contact lenses, watches, and rings. Then, in a quiet place where you will not be distracted for at least 30 minutes (and in the presence of soothing music if you choose), proceed as outlined below. Each session should take between 20 and 30 minutes and should be done at least once a day, with twice a day—once in the morning and once in the evening—being even better. Best performed to prevent headaches from occurring in the first place, the technique also can be employed to abort headaches once in progress. The

(continued on next page)

(continued)

technique also can be an effective aid to sleep if done just before retiring.

✔ Lie down on your back, either on the floor or on a good firm mattress, with a pillow under your head and/or your knees. Allow your breathing to become deep and even for about 10 seconds, then inhale and hold your breath as you:

✔ Lift your right arm perpendicular to the floor and gradually tense it to approximately 75 percent of maximum. Hold it in this contracted state for five seconds, then exhale as you slowly let it return to the floor, concentrating for the next 30 seconds on how warm and relaxed it now feels. Repeat this contraction-relaxation sequence twice more, then do the same with your left arm.

✔ Now repeat this same basic procedure, first with the muscle groups of your legs (raising each one approximately two feet from the floor and pointing your toes as you perform the five-second flex), your abdomen (arching your lower back slightly as you flex), your shoulders and back (curling up and looking at your feet as you flex), and finally your face (making the most grotesque expressions imaginable as you flex).

The purpose of these exercises, remember, is to impress on you the difference between how muscles feel in their contracted and relaxed states, so focus on this difference as intently as possible. The rationale behind the exercise is that once you are more alert to the difference, you will be better able to recognize when you may be tensing certain muscles involuntarily during moments of emotional stress—and then relax them accordingly.

■ The Relaxation Response

If the above procedure seems a bit involved for you, you might try this shorter and less-physical relaxation technique (at least daily) to help prevent stress-induced headaches. Developed by Herbert Benson, M.D., an associate professor of medicine at Harvard Medical School's Mind/Body Clinic, the exercise is

(continued on next page)

(continued)

designed to relax you in many of the same ways achieved by more arduous disciplines, such as transcendental meditation, yoga, and Zen.

While sitting quietly in a comfortable chair and breathing slowly and deeply, repeat a word or short phrase that has a special meaning to you. Repeat it every time you exhale. Don't worry if the image behind the phrase slips out of mind, but do bring it back if it does. The purpose of the exercise, in fact, is to help you master the mental control required for such retrieval. It's a strength you will later be able to employ to bring back peaceful thoughts during times of headache-producing stress. Practice the technique as often as three times a day, if you have the time, for at least 20 minutes per session.

■ Meditation

Meditation is a process similar to the Relaxation Response described above, in which you repeat to yourself a special sound or phrase (mantra) while sitting with your eyes closed and letting your mind wander. To learn the technique properly, however, taking a course in a specific approach to the discipline, called transcendental meditation, usually is advised.

■ Biofeedback

Best taught by a trained therapist, biofeedback is a process by which you learn to control normally involuntary bodily actions (such as heart rate, blood pressure, and the workings of the digestive system) with the help of feedback you get from being monitored by an electronic device. (Especially effective for aborting headaches once in progress, biofeedback is discussed further in Chapter 3.)

■ Yoga

Often described as meditation through movement, yoga seeks to relax the body through an intricate series of exercises and stretches designed to bring emotional as well as physical peace to the body. Too involved for an adequate portrayal here, it's best learned from an instructor, book, or videotape.

3 Treatment

It is estimated that 9 out of 10 Americans suffer from headaches and, unfortunately, the totals appear to be growing: Studies show that the number of people seeking treatment for migraine headaches has increased by an alarming 60 percent in the past 10 years.

So what's a person to do for headache relief?

Let's start with a comprehensive collection of the safest and most effective drugs now available for treating headaches. Then we'll survey the most tried-and-true of drug-free therapies and home remedies, as well as mind-control strategies for "thinking" away headaches and hands-on techniques for literally getting "physical" with your headache woes.

Treating Headaches With Drugs

There are hundreds of medications now available, prescription and nonprescription alike, that attack headaches. And they do it in a variety of ways. Some, termed *abortive*, include over-the-counter analgesics, such as aspirin and acetaminophen, which stop or reduce headaches by numbing the body's ability to feel pain. Others, termed *prophylactic*, are available by prescription only and work by treating the biological or emotional conditions responsible for causing headaches in the first place.

Start by seeing your family physician. You may need to see a headache specialist after that.

R. Michael Gallagher, D.O., secretary of the National Headache Foundation and professor and vice dean of the University of Medicine and Dentistry of New Jersey, explains: "Once considered an orphan disease because no one particular type of medical practice was being dedicated specifically to it, the problem of headaches now is being addressed by a variety of medical practitioners—family doctors, internists, neurologists, doctors of osteopathy, and even some dentists."

If your current physician is not able to treat your headache successfully, ask her to refer you to a specialist. Or contact the National Headache Foundation, Gallagher says. In addition to providing you with a list of over 1,400 member physicians nationwide specializing in the treatment of headaches, the nonprofit organization publishes a quarterly newsletter, provides educational programs on headaches, and offers free advice on headache problems. (To be approved for NHF membership, physicians must have their NHF applications, curriculum vitae, and state licenses approved by two other physician members; plus they must pay annual dues.)

The National Headache Foundation can be reached by writing 5252 North Western Avenue, Chicago, IL 60625 or by calling toll-free 800-843-2256.

 Don't take any medication for recurring headaches until you've consulted with your doctor.

There are so many types of headache medications that work in so many different ways that it is vital to find out which is the most appropriate for your specific headache frequency and type. Regular use (more than two days a week) of any medication designed for headache relief—and especially those containing caffeine—risks producing the rebound headaches we discussed in Chapter 2, as well as other potentially adverse side effects. If your headaches are occurring more than twice a week, for that matter, you probably are a candidate for a medication of a preventive rather than abortive nature, says the president of the National Headache Foundation, Robert S. Kunkel, M.D.

Rebound headaches are similar to the original headaches for which a medication is taken, Gallagher further explains, but may take on additional characteristics, such as shifts in pain location and increases in frequency and/or degree. As stated by Jerome Walker, M.D., in a report in the *Southern Medical Journal* (November 1993), overuse of headache medications may, in fact, be "the most common cause of chronic daily headaches suffered today."

 Use medication only as prescribed.

Regardless of whom you choose to treat your headache problems, do not make the mistake of negating his expertise by failing to follow medication or treatment guidelines, says Seymour Diamond, M.D., executive director of the National Headache Foundation and director of the Diamond Headache Clinic, Chicago. Do not vary the dosage or exceed recommended frequency of a medication without consulting your doctor. The balance between medication solving your headache problem or making it worse can be a delicate one. Following your practitioner's directions and working in partnership create an atmosphere that tends to produce better results.

A Comprehensive Guide to Headache Medications

If your headaches are relatively mild or do not occur more than twice a week, you may be a candidate for an analgesic or some other abortive type of medication designed to stop pain once it strikes. If your headaches are more severe, however, or occur more often than twice a week, you may be prescribed a prophylactic, or preventive, medication, meaning its purpose will be to treat the biological mechanisms suspected of causing your headaches in the first place.

Here's a rundown of what you need to know about the various types of headache medications currently available that fall into either of these abortive or prophylactic categories—prescription and nonprescription alike.

The "Abortives": Medications for Headache Relief

Remember, you probably are an appropriate candidate for medications of this type if your headaches occur two or fewer times a week.

 Don't consistently take any abortive medication for more than two days a week.

This applies to prescription and nonprescription abortive medications alike, the only exceptions being when headaches are so severe as to be incapacitating or they are suffered during a limited period, such as during illness or menstruation. Research indicates that as many as half of all chronic daily headaches may be due, in part, to overuse of the medications being taken to relieve them. Susceptibility to rebound headaches varies from person to person, but one study has shown that most people who fall prey to them are taking the pain-relieving equivalent of as few as three standard (325 mg.) aspirin tablets a day, reports Stephen D. Silberstein, M.D., clinical professor of neurology at Temple University School of Medicine, Philadelphia, and the scientific co-director of the American Association for the Study of Headache.

Writing in *Internal Medicine* (November 1993), Diamond says that to determine a patient's possible habituation to an analgesic, he inquires how long a bottle of 100 tablets lasts. "A patient may need detoxification if the bottle lasts less than one month."

 Know your abortive-medication options.

Should you take aspirin, acetaminophen, ibuprofen, naproxen sodium, or something more potent available by prescription only? That's a question you should discuss with your doctor, but here's an overview of the abortive medications currently meeting with the most success:

■ **Analgesics and analgesic combinations.** "Analgesics are appropriate for the treatment of infrequent, mild to moderate headaches, or very severe headaches unresponsive to more specific treatment," write Joel R. Saper, M.D., Stephen Silberstein, M.D., C. David Gordon,

M.D., and Robert L. Hamel in their *Handbook of Headache Management.** By the word "treatment," these doctors mean relief, not cure, however. Analgesics work not by correcting the biological cause of pain but rather by numbing the body's ability to perceive pain. So their use should not be thought of as curative in any way. They generally are safe and effective for the occasional relief of mild to moderate migraine and tension headaches alike, and come in both prescription and nonprescription forms. (See below.)

A word of caution regarding aspirin, however: Do not give aspirin or any medication containing salicylates to anyone 19 years of age or younger, unless directed by a physician, due to its association with Reye's syndrome, a potentially fatal condition. And regarding acetaminophen, this cautionary note from Glen Solomon, M.D., a headache specialist at the Cleveland Clinic Foundation and an associate professor

---

NONPRESCRIPTION ANALGESICS

(active ingredient amounts are per tablet or dose, if a liquid)

■ **Aspirin:** Bayer, Empirin (325 mg., except if otherwise specified)

■ **Aspirin plus buffers to reduce irritation to the stomach:** Bufferin, Ascriptin (325 mg., except if otherwise specified)

■ **Acetaminophen:** Tylenol, Datril, Panadol (325 mg.); Tempra, Liquiprin (liquid forms)

■ **Combination analgesics (those containing aspirin and/or acetaminophen in conjunction with caffeine to enhance absorption):** Excedrin (250 mg. aspirin, 250 mg. acetaminophen, 65 mg. caffeine); Vanquish (227 mg. aspirin, 194 mg. acetaminophen, 33 mg. caffeine plus buffers to reduce irritation to the stomach); Cope (421 mg. aspirin, 32 mg. caffeine plus buffers); Anacin (400 mg. aspirin, 32 mg. caffeine)

---

*Baltimore: Williams & Wilkins, 1993.

PRESCRIPTION ANALGESICS

As with nonprescription analgesics, prescription analgesics generally are effective for treating all types of headaches—migraine as well as tension-type—that occur two or fewer times a week. But they should not be used for headaches that occur more often than that. Check with your doctor regarding which of the following medications may be most suited for you given the specifics of your headaches and your overall health status.

■ **Combination analgesics containing barbiturates (potentially addictive sedatives that act on the central nervous system):** Fiorinal (325 mg. aspirin, 40 mg. caffeine, 50 mg. butalbital); Fioricet, Esgic (325 mg. acetaminophen, 40 mg. caffeine, 50 mg. butalbital); Phrenilin (325 mg. acetaminophen, 50 mg. butalbital)

■ **Combination analgesics containing codeine (a potentially addictive pain-relieving derivative of morphine):** Fiorinal with Codeine (325 mg. aspirin, 40 mg. caffeine, 50 mg. butalbital, 30 mg. codeine); Fioricet with Codeine (325 mg. acetaminophen, 50 mg. butalbital, 40 mg. caffeine, 30 mg. codeine); Tylenol Nos. 1/2/3/4 (325 mg. acetaminophen, 7.5/15/30/60 mg. codeine)

■ **Analgesics containing narcotics (potentially addictive pain relievers that act on the central nervous system):** Darvon (65 mg. propoxyphene HCL, 389 mg. aspirin, 323.4 mg. caffeine); Darvocet (50/100 mg. propoxyphene napsylate, 325 mg. acetaminophen); Vicodin (5 mg. hydrocodone, 500 mg. acetaminophen); Percocet (5 mg. oxycodone, 325 mg. acetaminophen); Percodan (4.5 mg. oxycodone, 325 mg. aspirin); Demerol (50/100 mg. meperidine)

of medicine at Ohio State University, Columbus: If you use acetaminophen and drink alcoholic beverages, do not mix the two. Instead, wait six hours to take acetaminophen after your last drink, or vice versa—that is, wait at least six hours after taking acetaminophen before having an alcoholic drink.

Be careful when taking any drug containing aspirin, as side effects can include rash, asthma, gastrointestinal irritation, and reduced blood coagulation. Also be aware of the dangers of acetaminophen, extended use of which (more than several months) may begin to cause kidney and liver damage, especially when taken in conjunction with alcohol. (See page 50.) Drawbacks to drugs containing narcotics include nausea, vomiting, sedation, respiratory depression, and dependence, and drugs containing barbiturates (also potentially addictive) may cause drowsiness.

All of the above drugs, for that matter, run the risk of making headaches worse rather than better if repeatedly used more than two days a week.

■ **Nonsteroidal Anti-Inflammatory Drugs (NSAIDs).** This category of medications relieves pain by reducing inflammation within tissues as well as by inhibiting the production of prostaglandins, substances that make you more sensitive to pain. Available in both prescription and nonprescription forms (see below), NSAIDs are effective for relieving both migraine and tension headaches of mild to moderate intensity. But these drugs should be used with caution by anyone suffering from stomach ulcers, colitis, gastritis, kidney disease, severe high blood pressure, bleeding disorders, or aspirin-sensitive asthma.

Side effects of NSAIDs may include gastrointestinal ulcers, mouth ulcers, colitis aggravation, sleepiness, and tinnitus (ringing in the ears).

Nonprescription (brand names in parentheses)
✔ ibuprofen (Medipren, Midol, Motrin, Nuprin)
✔ naproxen sodium (Alleve)

Prescription
✔ fenoprofen (Nalfon)
✔ naproxen (Naprosyn)
✔ ketoprofen (Orudis)
✔ indomethacin (Indocin)
✔ meclofenamate sodium (Meclomen)

✔ diclofenac sodium (Voltaren)
✔ piroxicam (Feldene)
✔ ketorolac (Toradol)
✔ sulindac (Clinoril)
✔ tolmetin (Tolectin)

■ **Ergotamine derivatives.** Ergotamine, or ergot, derivatives are the drugs of first choice for treating moderate to severe migraine and related headaches, according to Gallagher. Also effective against cluster headaches, they work by helping painfully swollen blood vessels of the head to return to normal. They may also help bring relief by reducing inflammation of the trigeminal nerve (see Chapter 1), which plays a critical role in many headaches. Available by prescription only, these medications should not be used during pregnancy or breast-feeding, nor should they be used by anyone with moderate to severe high blood pressure, stomach ulcers, heart problems, vascular disease, liver or kidney disease, or severe pruritus (itchy skin). Side effects may include nausea, vomiting, muscle cramps, angina, and paresthesia (itching and tingling of the skin). The following are brand names of the most common ergotamine derivatives currently being prescribed in the United States:

- ✔ Wigraine (available in tablet and suppository forms)
- ✔ Ergomar (available in tablet, suppository, and inhalant forms)
- ✔ Ergostat (available in tablet form)
- ✔ D.H.E. 45 (available in injectable form)
- ✔ Cafergot (available in suppository form)

■ **Isometheptene.** Isometheptene, the principal pain-relieving ingredient in Midrin and Isocom, is considered a good alternative for sufferers of moderate to severe migraine headaches who cannot tolerate ergotamine derivatives. It works as a vasoconstrictor and may be used in conjunction with NSAIDs for an even greater pain-relieving effect. The drug should not, however, be used by anyone suffering from glaucoma, liver or kidney disease, heart disease, or high blood pressure, and it may cause dizziness or sedation.

■ **Corticosteroids (generic examples: prednisone, hydrocortisone, methylprednisolone, dexamethasone).** Best reserved for circumstances in which other medications have failed, corticosteroids can be especially effective against cluster headaches and chronic and highly resistant migraines. Corticosteroids should not be taken in conjunction with aspirin or any other nonsteroidal anti-inflammatory drug, nor should they be taken during pregnancy or in the presence of infection or peptic ulcer. Side effects may include osteoporosis (with prolonged use), aggravation of diabetes and high blood pressure, myopathy (a disease of the muscles), Cushing's syndrome (a disease of the pituitary gland), and dependency.

■ **Sumatriptan (Imitrex).** The most recent weapon in the headache wars, sumatriptan was found effective in relieving migraine headaches in over 70 percent of patients in a study reported in the *New England Journal of Medicine* (August 1, 1991). A vasoconstrictor also effective in relieving cluster headaches, the drug appears relatively free of side effects and has the advantage over other migraine medications of being effective even when taken late in a migraine attack.

The "Prophylactics": Medications for Headache Prevention

 Know your prophylactic-medication options.

Are you a candidate for a medication of this type? You'll want to discuss this question with your doctor, of course, but here, according to the doctors who wrote *Handbook of Headache Management*, are the primary indicators that you may be a candidate for a preventive medication:

■ Your headaches occur more than two times a week.

■ Your headaches are debilitatingly severe.

■ Medications taken for symptomatic relief of your headaches have ceased to work.

■ Medications for symptomatic relief of your headaches are inadvisable due to their incompatibility with other medications you're taking for some other health problem.

■ Your doctor feels preventive medication may make medications taken for temporary symptomatic relief more effective.

If your doctor decides you are a candidate for a preventive medication, here are the types she's likely to offer:

■ **Beta-adrenergic blockers (generic examples: acebutolol, atenolol, esmolol, labetalol, metoprolol, nadolol, pindolol, propranolol, timolol).** These drugs are the medications of first choice for preventing migraine and other chronic vascular-type headaches, according to R. Michael Gallagher, D.O. (Research has shown them to be effective in reducing headache frequency in 60 to 80 percent of patients by at least 50 percent, report Saper, Silberstein, Gordon, and Hamel.) First developed for the treatment of heart problems like irregular heartbeat, angina pectoris, and high blood pressure, the drugs soon were discovered to be effective in preventing migraines. The drugs work relatively safely, by preventing the dilation of cranial arteries as well as by reducing blood-platelet aggregation, Seymour Diamond, M.D., explains. But they still may pose health risks for people suffering from asthma, congestive heart failure, diabetes, low blood sugar, low blood pressure, slow heartbeat, high blood fats, or vascular disease, according to research.

Side effects to be aware of, moreover, include fatigue, depression, memory disturbances, impotence, reduced tolerance for physical activity, decreases in blood pressure and heart rate, elevations in blood fats, bronchospasm, and weight gain.

■ **Calcium channel antagonists (generic examples: nifedipine, nimodipine, nicardipine, verapamil, diltiazem).** Slightly less effective in preventing migraine headaches than beta-adrenergic blockers yet more effective in treating cluster headaches (verapamil, especially), calcium channel antagonists are recommended for patients with some of the conditions that make beta-adrenergic blockers ill-advised— asthma, diabetes, high blood fats, and low blood sugar, for example. The drugs work by reducing inflammation of vascular nerves as well as by preventing vascular contraction, and while safe for most people, they do pose risks for people suffering from congestive heart failure, heart block, arterial flutter or fibrillation, low blood pressure, slow heart rate, sinus problems, or severe constipation, according to Saper, Silberstein, Gordon, and Hamel.

Side effects may include some of these same conditions— constipation, low blood pressure, and decreased heart rate, for example. Research shows that sleepiness, dizziness, nausea, and weight gain also may occur.

■ **Tricyclic antidepressants (generic examples: amitriptyline, nortriptyline, doxepin, desipramine, protriptyline).** Traditionally known for their efficacy in treating emotional disorders related to depression, tricyclic antidepressants more and more are becoming part of the arsenal of medications used to treat migraine headaches, and with good success, Gallagher reports. The drugs combat migraines in much the same biochemical way as they combat depressive disorders—by helping to stabilize blood levels of the brain chemical serotonin. (Shortages of serotonin are thought to be responsible for the painful vascular expansion of a migraine attack.) Not surprisingly, this stabilizing effect often makes antidepressants especially effective in preventing headaches due in part to a depressed emotional state, says Gallagher.

They have been found to be effective in preventing neck and face pain and pain syndromes related to sleep disturbances and anxiety, as well.

"Some patients express concern over being prescribed a psychiatric drug when they're suffering only from a physical problem," Gallagher concedes. "But this fear is an unwarranted one given both the pharmacology of these drugs and the lack of complications their use has encountered." Dosages generally are much smaller for the treatment of headaches, and the side effects of these drugs are minimal, even when they are prescribed in greater amounts for depression. "Certain precautions with tricyclic antidepressants, nonetheless, should be taken," Gallagher says. They need to be used with caution by anyone suffering from significant cardiac arrhythmia, low blood pressure, or glaucoma, and their side effects may include tremor, dizziness, confusion, restlessness, blurred vision, rapid heart rate, constipation, urinary retention, dry mouth, drowsiness, weight gain, and priapism (prolonged periods of penile erection).

■ **Fluoxetine (brand name Prozac).** Fluoxetine is a relatively recent nontricyclic antidepressant that has been shown to be effective in reducing the frequency and severity of most types of headaches. It also helps facial pain and pain related to psychiatric disturbances. As with tricyclic antidepressants, fluoxetine works by helping to stabilize serotonin (tricyclics do it by making cells more receptive to serotonin while fluoxetine helps prevent serotonin depletion in the first place). Fluoxetine generally entails fewer side effects than are common with tricyclic antidepressants, but its use warrants caution, nonetheless. It should not be used by anyone with a history of seizure disorders, and its side effects may include agitation, tremors, nausea, insomnia, diarrhea, and sexual dysfunction.

■ **MAO inhibitors (brand names Nardil, Parnate).** MAO (monoamine oxidase) inhibitors (MAOIs) are of best use against especially severe and resistant migraine headaches, severe and resistant chronic daily headaches and headaches in the presence of depression, obsessive-compulsive behavior, and panic disorder. Caffeine, alcohol, and foods high in tyramine content (see Chapter 2) should be avoided when MAOIs are being taken, and side effects can include the following: low blood pressure upon standing, high blood pressure when combined with a contraindicated food substance or drug, reduced sex drive, constipation, insomnia, water retention, and weight gain.

A word of caution: MAO inhibitors can be very effective, but because of their potential for adverse effects when taken in conjunction with foods high in tyramine and certain drugs (antidepressants, appetite suppressants, asthma medications, decongestants, nasal sprays, and anticonvulsants), they should be taken only under the supervision of a physician well experienced in their use.

■ **Ergotamine derivatives (generic examples: methysergide, methylergonovine).** Recommended for highly resistant migraines, menstrual migraines, chronic daily headaches, cluster headaches, and facial pain, these drugs can be highly effective. But because of their potential for causing numerous side effects and rebound headaches, they should be used only under the close supervision of a physician well experienced in their use. They should not be used during pregnancy or in the presence of high blood pressure, liver or kidney problems, cardiovascular disease, or phlebitis. Side effects may include nausea, aching muscles, hallucinations, and (in very rare cases) damage to the pancreas, gallbladder, and/or lungs.

■ **Anticonvulsants (generic examples: phenytoin, carbamazepine).** Although effective in the treatment of migraines, daily chronic headaches, cluster headaches, and facial pain, anticonvulsants can reduce the effectiveness of oral contraceptives and definitely should not be used during pregnancy because of significant risks of fetal deformity. Other adverse reactions may include dizziness, drowsiness, insomnia, rash, and lapses in muscular coordination. Anticonvulsants also can be toxic when used in conjunction with fluoxetine (Prozac).

■ **Antihistamines (generic examples: cyproheptadine, hydroxyzine).** These drugs are especially suited for the treatment of migraine headaches in children. Side effects may include sedation and weight gain.

■ **Lithium carbonate.** Best known for treating manic-depression, lithium has been shown to be effective in treating cluster headaches and migraines that occur on a cyclical basis. Side effects to be aware of include tremor, thirst, water retention, mental changes, and excessive urination.

12 Effective Alternative Therapies

"Although drugs have represented the mainstay of traditional headache treatments, it is important to try to find safer and equally effective means of relieving or preventing headaches," according to Diamond. "Stress, anxiety, and depression—all have the potential to be powerful headache triggers, hence any method that is effective in treating these emotional states has great potential for being effective as a headache palliative."

People preferring to avoid the unwanted side effects of drugs look to alternative methods of headache relief. Disciplines include therapies to relax the body, some by relaxing the mind and others by relaxing both. What follows is a roundup of nonmedicinal therapies that research shows have been meeting with the most success.

Getting Physical

Headaches may be felt primarily in the head, but muscular tension and stiffness within the body can be the source of this pain. Relief for many headaches can be as close as the massaging action of your own fingertips. Here, according to various headache experts, are some of the best ways to "get physical" with your headache woes—techniques that can be performed, moreover, with the help of no one other than yourself!

 Press your pain away.

Because parts of the body are more intimately connected than we sometimes realize, pressing on some areas can have effects on other areas distantly removed, says Fred D. Sheftell of the New England

Center for Headache, Stamford, Connecticut. A pressing action employs the basic principle of the ancient Chinese art of acupressure, which maintains that pain sometimes is caused by blocked nerve impulses at various key sites throughout the body. Exerting pressure at these sites helps clear the blockages, thus restoring proper "neurological flow."

For the relief of headaches, try pressing or squeezing at one or more of the following sites for approximately 20 seconds, Sheftell says. Release for 10 seconds, then repeat four times.

Areas to try: the web of skin between your thumb and forefinger; the top of your foot between your big and middle toes; the area outside your shinbone just below your knee; the Achilles tendon at the back of your heel; your temples; two spots at the right and left of your spinal column at the base of your skull at a level even with your earlobes.

 ### Rub or brush your pain away.

Another hands-on approach to headaches is a good, firm massage, says orthopedic surgeon David F. Fardon, M.D., author of *Free Yourself From Neck Pain and Headache*. More suitable for tension headaches than for vascular headaches like migraines, massaging the scalp can help flush away pain by restoring blood flow to areas being shortchanged of blood due to tense muscles. (In migraine headaches, remember, excessive blood flow is the cause of pain.)

You can implement this flushing action either by massaging your forehead, neck, and scalp with your fingertips (as if washing your hair) or using a hairbrush with firm bristles. If you're using your fingertips, "begin over your forehead and apply deep pressure, making small circles," Fardon says. Slowly direct this massaging action to your temples, then above your ears, and finally down the muscles of the back of your neck and into your shoulders. If you choose to use a hairbrush, follow this same path and employ the same circular action.

Chase the hurt with heat.

Another way of stepping up sluggish blood flow through the blood vessels of the head and scalp, and hence relieving tension headaches, is to apply heat to these areas, says headache specialist Glen Solomon of the Cleveland Clinic. The restored blood flow replenishes oxygen to "suffocating" muscles as it also helps flush away the accumulation of pain-producing toxins.

To achieve these benefits, place a heating pad at the back of your head for 20 to 30 minutes, Solomon says. Or for an even more penetrating heat, take a long hot shower with the spray directed at the back of your neck, or a hot bath with your head and neck emersed as much as possible. (As dizziness and changes in blood pressure may result, especially from the latter self-care treatment, consult with your practitioner first.)

 ## Ease the ache with ice.

If you're suffering from a vascular headache, your problem is not a shortage but rather a surplus of blood flowing through the blood vessels of your head and scalp. Hence the wisdom of ice. By applying ice to these areas, you cause blood vessels to constrict, thereby reducing blood flow and the pain associated with it, explains Sheftell. He recommends an ice pack wrapped in a towel for this purpose, or a pack of frozen vegetables, or a specially designed ice pillow (available at most drugstores). Place the cold pack at your forehead or on the top of your head at the earliest sign of headache onset, Sheftell says.

 ## Try acupuncture.

Acupuncture reportedly was inspired by the observation by Chinese healers back before the birth of Christ that soldiers wounded with arrows sometimes experienced relief from diseases that had been troubling them for years. The discipline subsequently evolved into a detailed system whereby various physical ills were treated by penetrating the skin at specific points with the use of extremely sharp needles. The practice continues today, in the hands of licensed acupuncturists, many of whom also have degrees in conventional medicine. Though the efficacy of the practice remains in question, one British study found that 80 percent of chronic headache sufferers experienced total cure or considerable improvement after acupuncture, despite meeting with no success at all after being treated by at least two other doctors.

Check with your doctor or local hospital or health center for a licensed practitioner in your area.

 ## Try wearing a headband.

Fashion aside, tying a cloth or scarf tightly around the head can help relieve a headache (if it's a migraine) by reducing blood flow to the scalp, which is in painful abundance during a migraine attack. In a 1992 study, researchers at the University of California at Davis School of Medicine reported that use of an elastic headband by 23 migraine sufferers was found to reduce most of their headaches by at least 80 percent. (Their headaches did return, however, when the band was removed.)

 ## Upgrade your lighting.

In addition to excessive blood flow to the head and scalp, sometimes eyestrain can cause headaches, and there's no greater cause of that than inadequate light, says Robert A. Baron, Ph.D., an industrial psychologist and professor at the Rensselaer Polytechnic Institute, in Troy, New York. Fluorescent lighting can be especially exhausting for the eyes, he says, because though it may appear to be "on" constantly, it actually flickers about 60 times a second. If you have fluorescent lights in your home or workplace, try replacing them with conventional incandescent bulbs, Baron suggests. You just may "black-out" some of your headaches if you do.

 ## Seek seclusion.

"Probably the simplest thing you can do to relieve a headache is to go into a dark, quiet room and lie down," says Solomon. This is because movement of any kind can aggravate many headaches, as can light and noise. Retreat to your bedroom, loosen any tight clothing and remove your shoes, close the curtains and douse the lights – and let the blissful silence do the rest.

Getting Mental

Just as the body can be a worthy focus for achieving the relaxation needed to relieve headaches, so can the mind – the place where stress and anxiety often begin their assaults on our health in the first place. Here are the mental techniques currently being employed most successfully in headache treatment.

 ## "Visualize" your pain away.

"In general terms, visualization is a technique whereby the body's own healing mechanisms are stimulated by conjuring in the mind images of positive and pleasant objects or scenes," explains Jenny Sutcliffe in *The Complete Book of Relaxation Techniques.**

Sound like wishful thinking? Donna Copeland, Ph.D., a clinical psychologist and president of the American Psychological Association's Division of Psychological Hypnosis, says visualization can be "a very effective tool for dealing with pain and anxiety."

---

* Allentown, Pa.: People's Medical Society, 1994.

Learning the technique with a trained professional is best, but Copeland says many people, if they really put their minds to it, can achieve significant results on their own. The next time you feel a headache coming on, remove yourself to a quiet place, sit or lie down, close your eyes, and imagine as vividly as possible one or more of the following scenes:

■ See yourself diving into a warm ocean surf off a beautiful white sandy beach.

■ Imagine yourself standing atop a snow-crested mountain breathing cool, fresh air.

■ Picture yourself relaxing peacefully in a warm, bubbling hot tub.

If you can conjure images even more soothing than these, do so. Whatever scenario is most personally relaxing for you is going to have the greatest tranquilizing effect.

 Escape pain "autogenically."

Developed by German psychiatrist Johannes Schults in the 1930s, autogenic therapy seeks to achieve pain relief by relaxing the body using specific mental commands designed to attain a semihypnotic state. According to Seymour Diamond, M.D., most reputable headache clinics have these therapists on staff.

Best taught by a licensed practitioner, the technique can, however, be learned by do-it-yourselfers capable of sufficient concentration. If you think that's you, here's how to proceed:

■ Lie down in a quiet spot where you will not be disturbed.

■ Breathe deeply and begin repeating the following phrases under your breath until the effect of each is achieved:
    ✔ "My legs and arms are heavy."
    ✔ "My legs and arms are warm."
    ✔ "My heart is steady and calm."
    ✔ "My breathing is steady and calm."
    ✔ "My abdomen is relaxed and warm."
    ✔ "My forehead is cool and clear."

■ Once all of these states have been reached, keep repeating the final phrase while keeping your fingers crossed as a physical confirmation of what you've achieved. The entire exercise should take approximately 30 minutes and be done no fewer than three times a week, or whenever headaches strike.

Getting Electric

 Learn to relax with biofeedback.

Useful for relieving tension and vascular headaches alike, biofeedback is a technique whereby an electronic device is used to monitor physical signs of emotional stress (heart rate, blood pressure, or muscular tension) so that relaxation can be learned on a biological level. The technique is best learned from a trained professional in a clinical setting, but once mastered, the practice can be continued with biofeedback machines that have been developed for use at home.

In the treatment of tension headaches, small electrodes capable of measuring muscular tension are attached to the temples. When muscular tension is high, the biofeedback machine emits high-pitched tones. When muscular tension decreases, the tone lowers, thus permitting the biofeedback participant an immediately discernible measure of the degree of muscular relaxation being achieved. The intent of the procedure is that the patient will learn to relax without the help of the machine, and research demonstrates considerable success. Studies done at the Diamond Headache Clinic in Chicago, for example, found the procedure to be effective in reducing headache severity, duration, and frequency in 68 percent of patients trained in the technique.

 Try TENS *to terminate a headache.*

Used to treat back, neck, joint and muscular pain as well as headaches, TENS (transcutaneous electrical nerve stimulation) is a technique that uses alternating, low-voltage electrical current to abort pain by eliciting the production of endorphins (natural painkillers) while also blocking the transmission of nerve impulses. Electrodes are attached to the skin in the area where pain is being experienced, then pulsating electrical current is transmitted via these electrodes. Within 30 minutes, considerable pain reduction—although temporary in most cases—usually is enjoyed.

Recently an updated version of TENS using direct rather than alternating current was tested by researchers from Sri Ramachandra Medical College, in India, with encouraging results. Whereas all but 2 of 48 patients who had experienced relief from daily TENS treatments experienced a return of their headaches within two days when treatments were stopped, all 47 patients in the direct-current group saw their pain relief last at least six months.

TENS machines are available for home use, but receiving the therapy from a trained professional, at least initially, is advised. Check with your family doctor or local hospital or medical care center for names of professionals in your area. (Many chiropractors now offer TENS, too.)

So there you have it: a variety of suggestions, both therapeutic and preventive, for stopping the pain of headaches. True, not every method will work for everybody, but you can custom-design your own program. Sample these tips until you find the ones that work best for you. And remember, considerable and often complete relief is attainable.

■ APPENDIX

The Complete Headache Chart

■ Tension-Type Headaches

Symptoms: Dull, nonthrobbing pain, frequently bilateral, associated with tightness of scalp or neck. Degree of severity remains constant.

Precipitating Factors: Emotional stress. Hidden depression.

Treatment: Rest, aspirin, acetaminophen, ibuprofen, naproxen sodium, combinations of analgesics with caffeine, ice packs, muscle relaxants. Antidepressants if appropriate, biofeedback, psychotherapy. If necessary, *temporary* use of stronger prescription analgesics.

Prevention: Avoidance of stress. Use of biofeedback, relaxation techniques, or antidepressant medication.

■ Migraine Without Aura

Symptoms: Severe, one-sided throbbing pain, often accompanied by nausea, vomiting, cold hands, tremor, dizziness, sensitivity to sound, and light.

Precipitating Factors: Certain foods. Use of the Pill or hormone replacement therapy. Excessive hunger, change in altitude or weather. Bright or flashing lights. Excessive smoking, emotional stress. Hereditary component.

Treatment: Ice packs. Analgesics such as aspirin, acetaminophen, or ibuprofen. Medications known as vasoconstrictors, such as ergotamine, which constrict the blood vessels. Sumatriptan is available for subcutaneous self-injection. The non-steroidal anti-inflammatory agents (NSAIDs) may also be helpful. For prolonged attacks, steroids may be helpful.

Prevention: Avoidance of precipitating factors. Biofeedback. Propranolol. The calcium channel blockers and the NSAIDs may help prevent migraine headaches.

■ Migraine With Aura

Symptoms: Same as for migraine without aura, except victim develops warning symptoms. These may include visual disturbances, numbness in arm or leg, the smelling of strange odors, hallucinations. Preliminary reaction subsides within one-half hour and is followed by severe pain.

Precipitating Factors: Same as migraine without aura.

Treatment: At earliest onset of symptoms, use of biofeedback, ergotamine, or sumatriptan. Once pain has begun, treatment is the same as for migraine without aura.

Prevention: Same as migraine without aura.

■ Cluster Headaches

Symptoms: Excruciating pain around or behind one eye. Tearing of eye, congestion of nose, flushing of face. Pain frequently develops during sleep and may last for several hours. Attacks occur every day for weeks or months, then disappear for up to a year. Ninety percent of cluster patients are male, most between ages 20 and 30.

Precipitating Factors: Alcoholic beverages, excessive smoking.

Treatment: Ergotamine or oxygen inhalation. Intranasal application of local anesthetic agent.

Prevention: Steroids, ergotamine, methysergide. Small regular doses of lithium carbonate for chronic cluster headaches.

■ Menstrual Headaches

Symptoms: Migraine-type pain that occurs shortly before, during, or after menstruation or mid-cycle, at time of ovulation.

Precipitating Factors: Variance in estrogen levels.

Treatment: Same as for migraine.

Prevention: Small doses of vasoconstrictors before and during menstrual period. Anti-inflammatory drugs during menstruation may also help.

■ Hypertension Headaches

Symptoms: Generalized or "hatband" type pain, most severe in morning. Diminishes as day goes on.

Precipitating Factors: Severe hypertension: over 200 systolic and 110 diastolic.

Treatment: Appropriate blood-pressure medication.

Prevention: Keep blood pressure under control.

■ Aneurysm

Symptoms: Early symptoms may mimic frequent migraine or cluster headaches. Cause is balloonlike weakness or bulge in blood-vessel wall. May rupture or allow blood to leak slowly. A ruptured aneurysm (stroke) results in sudden, unbearable headache, double vision, rigid neck. Victim rapidly becomes unconscious.

Precipitating Factors: Cogenital tendency. Extreme hypertension.

Treatment: If diagnosed early, surgery.

Prevention: Keep blood pressure under control.

■ Sinus Headaches

Symptoms: A gnawing pain over nasal area, often increasing in severity as day goes on. Caused by acute infection, usually with fever, producing blockage of sinus ducts and preventing normal drainage. Sinus headaches are rare—migraine and cluster headaches are often misdiagnosed as sinus in origin.

Precipitating Factors: Infection, nasal polyps, anatomical deformities, such as deviated septum, that block the sinus ducts.

Treatment: Antibiotics, decongestants, surgical drainage if necessary.

Prevention: None.

■ Hangover Headaches

Symptoms: Migrainelike symptoms of throbbing pain and nausea.

Precipitating Factors: Alcohol, which causes dilation and irritation of the blood vessels of the brain and surrounding tissue.

Treatment: Liquids (including broth). Consumption of fructose (honey and tomato juice are good sources) to help burn alcohol.

Prevention: Drink only in moderation.

■ Allergy Headaches

Symptoms: Nasal congestion, watery eyes.

Precipitating Factors: Seasonal allergens, such as pollen, molds. Allergies to food are *not* usually a factor.

Treatment: Antihistamine medication or desensitization injections.

Prevention: Desensitization.

■ Caffeine-Withdrawal Headaches

Symptoms: Throbbing headache caused by rebound dilation of the blood vessels several hours after consumption of large quantities of caffeine.

Precipitating Factors: Caffeine.

Treatment: Stop caffeine consumption.

Prevention: Avoidance of caffeine.

■ Exertional Headaches

Symptoms: Generalized head pain during or following physical exertion (as in running, jumping, or sexual intercourse) or passive exertion (sneezing, coughing, moving one's bowels, etc.).

Precipitating Factors: Organic diseases, such as aneurysms, tumors, or blood-vessel malformation, are the precipitating factors in about 10 percent of exertional headaches. The rest are usually related to migraine or cluster headaches already in progress. Cause *must* be accurately determined.

Treatment: Most commonly aspirin, indomethacin, or propranolol. Surgery to correct organic disease is occasionally indicated.

Prevention: None.

■ Trauma Headaches

Symptoms: Localized or generalized pain, can mimic migraine symptoms. Headaches usually occur on daily basis and are frequently resistant to treatment.

Precipitating Factors: Pain can occur after relatively minor trauma. Cause of pain is often difficult to diagnose.

Treatment: Possible help from anti-inflammatory drugs, propranolol, biofeedback.

Prevention: Standard precautions against trauma.

■ Hunger Headaches

Symptoms: Pain, which strikes just before mealtime, caused by muscle tension, low blood sugar, and rebound dilation of the blood vessels.

Precipitating Factors: Strenuous dieting or skipping meals.

Treatment: Regular, nourishing meals containing adequate protein and complex carbohydrates.

Prevention: Same as treatment.

■ Temporomandibular Joint (TMJ) Headaches

Symptoms: A muscle-contraction type of pain, sometimes accompanied by a "clicking" sound on opening the jaw. Infrequent cause of headache.

Precipitating Factors: Malocclusion (poor bite), stress, and jaw clenching.

Treatment: Relaxation, biofeedback, use of bite plate. In extreme cases correction of malocclusion.

Prevention: Same as treatment.

■ Tic Douloureux Headaches

Symptoms: Short, jablike pain in facial area, often around the mouth or jaw. Pain lasts from several seconds to several months. Can occur many times a day. Relatively rare disease of the neural impulses; more common in women after age 55.

Precipitating Factors: Cause unknown. Pain brought on by chewing, cold air, even touching face. If condition occurs under age 55, neurological disease, such as MS, may be a factor.

Treatment: Anticonvulsants and muscle relaxants. Neurosurgery.

Prevention: None.

■ Fever Headaches

Symptoms: Generalized head pain that develops with fever. Caused by inflammation of the blood vessels of the head.

Precipitating Factors: Infection.

Treatment: Aspirin, acetaminophen, antibiotics.

Prevention: None.

■ Arthritis Headaches

Symptoms: Pain at back of head or neck. Intensifies on movement. Inflammation of joints and muscles.

Precipitating Factors: Unknown.

Treatment: Anti-inflammatory drugs. Muscle relaxants.

Prevention: None.

■ Eyestrain Headaches

Symptoms: Usually frontal, bilateral pain, directly related to using eyes. Rare cause of headache.

Precipitating Factors: Muscle imbalance. Uncorrected vision, astigmatism.

Treatment: Correction of vision.

Prevention: Same as treatment.

■ Temporal Arteritis

Symptoms: A boring, burning, or jabbing pain caused by inflammation of the temporal arteries. Pain, often around ear, on chewing. Weight loss, problems with eyesight. Rare: affects people over 50.

Precipitating Factors: Cause unknown. May be due to immune disorder.

Treatment: Steroids.

Prevention: None.

■ Tumor Headaches

Symptoms: Symptoms include pain that becomes progressively worse; projectile vomiting; possible visual disturbances; speech or personality changes; problems with equilibrium, gait, or coordination; seizures. Condition is extremely rare.

Precipitating Factors: Usually unknown.

Treatment: Surgery and/or radiation.

Prevention: None.

Used with permission, National Headache Foundation, 5252 North Western Avenue, Chicago, IL 60625; 800-843-2256.

■ GLOSSARY

Acupressure (shiatsu): A form of deep massage developed from the principles of acupuncture. Fingers rather than needles are used to relieve pain and promote health by restoring the flow of neurological energy along special neurological pathways called meridians.

Acupuncture: An ancient Chinese method of controlling pain and curing disease in which needles are inserted into the skin at certain strategic points along special neurological pathways (called meridians) for the purpose of restoring the proper flow of neurological energy.

Amines: Biological substances produced by the body, but also found in some foods, that play a role in headaches by affecting blood-vessel expansion and contraction.

Analgesics: Medications ranging from simple aspirin and acetaminophen to stronger drugs like codeine and morphine. Analgesics reduce pain by blocking the transmission of pain impulses. They do nothing to affect the biological causes of pain.

Aneurysm: A weakness in a blood-vessel wall that results in a bulge that can rupture and cause hemorrhaging if not treated in time.

Antidepressants: Medications that help restore shortages of brain chemicals thought to be responsible for depressive disorders as well as the headaches that frequently accompany such disturbed emotional states. Antidepressants also can be effective in treating headaches not accompanied by depression.

Arteritis: A swelling condition of the walls of one or more arteries.

Arthritis: A chronic condition, characterized by inflammation within joints, that can produce headaches when occurring in the areas of the neck and cervical spine.

Aura: A 10- to 30-minute period of sensory disturbances (often including blurred vision, flashing lights, tingling of the skin, dizziness, lack of muscle control, and mental confusion) that precedes the headache phase of a migraine attack in some migraine sufferers.

Barbiturates: A class of drugs that work on the central nervous system to act as sedatives or induce sleep.

Beta-adrenergic blockers: A group of medications helpful in preventing stress-related migraine headaches by blocking the effects of adrenaline on the expansion and contraction of blood vessels.

Biofeedback: A method of relaxation effective in relieving headaches. In biofeedback, a person learns to control such involuntary actions as heart rate and blood pressure with the help of an electronic device that monitors these functions.

Caffeine: A chemical substance occurring naturally in coffee, tea, cola drinks, and chocolate and also added to certain headache analgesics; helps to abort headaches by causing painfully expanded blood vessels to constrict.

Chinese restaurant syndrome: A condition named for the presence in many Chinese foods of monosodium glutamate (MSG), which is known to cause headaches and sweating in some people by expanding blood vessels in the areas of the head and face.

Classic migraine: A type of migraine headache (affecting a small percentage of all migraine sufferers) in which the headache phase of the attack is preceded by 10 to 30 minutes of bizarre sensory disturbances called an aura.

Cluster headaches: Extremely painful vascular headaches so named for their proclivity for striking in groups of two or more within several hours, then disappearing for weeks or even years before striking again. Pain typically is experienced as an intense stabbing or burning sensation in or around one of the eyes accompanied by tearing of the affected eye, facial flushing, and nasal congestion.

Common migraine: A migraine headache similar to a classic migraine (exhibiting the same side effects of nausea and hypersensitivity to noise and light) but different by virtue of occurring without the premonitory phase of sensory disturbances called an aura.

Computerized axial tomography (CT, or CAT, scan): A technique for detecting organic causes of headaches that uses a computer to combine hundreds of x rays into a single picture capable of being analyzed far more accurately than single x rays.

Depression: A psychological disorder characterized by chronic feelings of dejection and hopelessness. Depression is thought to be a contributing factor in as many as half of all headaches suffered on a chronic basis.

Dihydroergotamine (DHE): An injectable form of ergotamine tartrate found very helpful in relieving cluster and severe migraine headaches without as many side effects as ergotamine tartrate, which is taken in oral form.

Encephalitis: An inflammation of the brain; usually caused by a viral infection that comes from the sting of a mosquito. Among its symptoms are headache and neck pain.

Endorphins: One of two pain-relieving substances produced naturally by the body and thought to be released in response to certain relaxation techniques as well as by physical exercise.

Enkephalins: One of two pain-relieving substances produced naturally by the body and thought to be released in response to certain relaxation techniques as well as by physical exercise.

Ergotamine tartrate: A drug (derived from the mold that grows on rye) that works especially well to relieve migraine headaches (classic as well as common) by causing swollen blood vessels on the surface of the brain to return to a more normal size.

Estrogen: Female hormone that is suspected of increasing the frequency, duration, and severity of migraine headaches, especially when taken in the form of birth-control pills or hormone-replacement therapy following menopause.

Exertional headaches: Headaches caused by the expansion of blood vessels of the muscles of the head, neck, and scalp in response to physical exertion and/or such actions as coughing, sneezing, or straining at stool.

Extracranial: Referring to anatomical structures (i.e., nerves, blood vessels, muscles) located outside the cranium, or skull.

Facial pain: Pain experienced by the nerves of the face due to triggers that also can cause migraines.

Glaucoma: A group of eye diseases capable of causing headaches due to a buildup of pressure within the eyes.

Histamine: A substance released by the body in response to cellular injury; considered a causative factor in cluster headaches as well as in migraines.

Hot-dog headache: A headache suffered in response to eating foods containing sodium nitrite, a preservative used to prevent the development of bacteria in cured meats like hot dogs, ham, salami, and bacon.

Hypertension (or **high blood pressure):** A possible cause of headaches if extreme – regularly higher than 200/110 mm/Hg.

Hypnosis: A method of headache relief in which a therapist puts the patient into a subconscious state and instructs him to forget the pain.

Hypoxia: A lack of oxygen accompanied by a surplus of carbon dioxide in the blood; suspected of triggering migraine headaches by causing a swelling of blood vessels in the brain.

Ice-cream headache: A headache brought on by irritation of the trigeminal nerve, which is located at the back of the throat, in response to rapidly consuming a food or beverage that's very cold.

Inflammation: Swelling, redness, and pain caused by a sudden influx of blood cells intended for repair into an area of injured tissue. Headaches, vascular as well as tension-type, can result when the inflammation caused by such an influx irritates nerves of the head, neck, face, scalp, or layer of padding (meninges) inside the skull.

Meningitis: Inflammation of the brain's protective coating (the meninges), caused by infection, that can produce headaches as long as the infection persists.

Menstruation: A common contributor to migraine headaches in many women due to hormonal changes responsible for increased levels of pain-sensitizing substances called prostaglandins.

Monosodium glutamate (MSG): A flavor enhancer prevalent in many Chinese and processed foods that can cause headaches as well as sweating and tightness in the chest, the result of inordinate vascular expansion in people sensitive to the compound.

Muscular-contraction headache (also called **tension headache**): Head pain due to irritation of nerves caused by prolonged contraction of muscles of the neck, shoulders, face, or scalp; usually infrequent, due to occasional periods of fatigue or stressful events. Tension headaches also can be chronic if caused by an ongoing psychological problem or depressive state.

Nicotine: A powerful vasoconstrictor capable of triggering both migraine and cluster headaches.

Nitrates: Potent vasodilators (found in many heart medications), these compounds are proven culprits in the onset of migraines and other headaches vascular in origin.

Nitrites: Potent vasodilators (used as preservatives in cured meats), these compounds are proven culprits in the onset of migraines and other headaches vascular in origin.

Placebo: A drug or treatment that, despite having no true medical benefits, produces positive results due purely to a patient's belief that it will. It has been estimated that as many as 30 percent of all people will exhibit a response of this type.

Platelet antagonists: A group of medications effective in treating migraine headaches by virtue of their ability to normalize serotonin levels by preventing blood platelets from clumping together.

Prostaglandins: Substances, released by various organs, thought to play a role in migraine headaches by encouraging blood-platelet aggregation and consequent overproduction of the vasoconstrictor serotonin.

Ptosis: Drooping of one of the eyelids characteristic of a cluster headache.

Referred pain: Pain experienced in one area of the body although caused by irritation of nerves elsewhere.

Scotoma: A blind spot in the field of vision common during the aura stage of a classic migraine attack; thought to be due to a temporary shortage of blood to the brain.

Serotonin: A potent constrictor of blood vessels suspected as a cause of cluster headaches and migraines; a substance found naturally in the brain and intestines.

Sinusitis: An infection of the linings of the sinus cavities that can result in headaches when accompanied by fever and blockage of the sinuses with pus.

Temporal arteritis: A swelling disorder of the blood vessels of the head, principally the temporal artery; most common in people over the age of 55 and characterized by headache that cannot be relieved.

Temporomandibular joint disorder (TMJ): A malfunctioning of the jaw, due to muscle or ligament strain or sometimes arthritis, that can cause head and face pain as well as a sensation of blockage in the ear. Relief is best achieved by applications of heat or, in more extreme cases, muscle relaxants or tranquilizers.

Tranquilizer: A drug that can help relieve headaches by reducing anxiety and emotional stress, but which can cause physical or mental addiction to the drug.

Transcutaneous electrical nerve stimulation (TENS): A method of pain control in which a mild electrical current is administered through electrodes attached to the skin with the intent of interrupting pain signals to the brain. It's believed by some researchers that the mild shocks also may increase the body's production of pain-relieving endorphins.

Trigeminal nerve: A major sensory nerve (which emerges from the brain at the base of the skull) responsible for carrying sensations to the brain from most portions of the face and scalp as well as from the thin layer of protective tissue (the meninges) that covers the brain.

Tumor: A benign or malignant mass of tissue that arises for no functional purpose from cells of preexistent tissue. When such a growth appears on the brain, headaches (experienced as a dull ache and typically made worse by coughing, sneezing, or physical exertion) can result from the pressure exerted by the tumor on nearby nerves. Other neurological symptoms, such as changes in handwriting, personality, or thought patterns, also may occur.

Tyramine: An amino acid, found in some foods and also produced by the body, that can trigger headaches by causing vasodilation in people sensitive to it.

Vasoconstriction: A narrowing of blood vessels; responsible for the aura stage of classic migraine headaches.

Vasodilation: An expansion of blood vessels; responsible for the headache phase of both classic and common migraine attacks.

Weather-related headache: Headache triggered by changes in climatic conditions, such as barometric pressure, humidity, wind velocity, and temperature.

■ INDEX